More Than Just a Meal

of related interest

Therapeutic Art Directives and Resources
Activities and Initiatives for Individuals and Groups
Susan R. Makin
Commentaries by Cathy Malchiodi
ISBN 1 85302 824 X

Contemporary Art Therapy with Adolescents
Shirley Riley
Forewords by Gerald D. Oster and Cathy Malchiodi
ISBN 1 85302 637 9 pb
ISBN 1 85302 636 0 hb

Self-Mutilation and Art Therapy
Violent Creation
Diana Milia
ISBN 1 85302 683 4

Arts Therapies and Clients with Eating Disorders
Fragile Board
Edited by Ditty Dokter
ISBN 1 85302 256 X

Anorexics on Anorexia
Edited by Rosemary Shelley
ISBN 1 85302 471 6

More Than Just a Meal

The Art of Eating Disorders

Susan R. Makin

Forewords by Bryan Lask and Cathy Malchiodi

Jessica Kingsley Publishers
London and Philadelphia

First published in the United Kingdom in 2000
by Jessica Kingsley Publishers
116 Pentonville Road
London N1 9JB, UK
and
400 Market Street, Suite 400
Philadelphia, PA 19106, USA

www.jkp.com

Library of Congress Cataloging in Publication Data
Makin, Susan R.
    More than just a meal : the art of eating disorders / Susan R. Makin.
        p.   cm.
    Includes bibliogrpahical references and index.
    ISBN 1 85302 805 3 (pbk. : alk paper)
    1. Eating disorders-- Treatment. 2. Art therapy. I. Title.
RC552.E18M34   1999   99-43182
616.85'2606515--dc21   CIP

British Library Cataloguing in Publication Data
A CIP catalogue record for this book is available from the British Library

ISBN-13: 978 1 85302 805 2
ISBN-10: 1 85302 805 3

Contents

List of Plates

List of Figures

List of Tables

Foreword

Bryan Lask

Eating disorders are difficult to understand, detrimental to both physical and psychological health, and extraordinarily difficult to treat. During the early stages of an eating disorder the client will not even be aware that she has a problem; and once this has become evident she will commonly refuse treatment. Indeed eating disorders are probably the only group of disorders in which the client does not want treatment. Consequently it can prove very problematic trying to engage in the treatment process. No one treatment has proved to be adequate and the more traditional psychotherapies are far from the client's liking.

Why then art therapy? The answer is succinctly supplied in the 'Testimony to art therapy' (p.15). The client who has difficulty in recognizing she has a problem, and even more difficulty in exploring and expressing those problems once they are recognized, may feel considerably more comfortable using art as a medium of exploration and expression. This applies throughout the age ranges, but particularly for children and adolescents with eating disorders.

Susan Makin's book, clearly, logically and sympathetically, helps us to understand eating disorders, art therapy, and their integration. For good measure she also introduces us to the way in which poetry therapy can be added to support the therapeutic process. Susan Makin takes us into the world of the client with an eating disorder, helps us to understand better the conflict, confusion and suffering, and shows how experiential and creative work can steer and guide to recovery. This is a book that can be dipped into or read from cover to cover; either way there is an enormous amount to be gained by the reader from the author's wisdom, empathy, clarity and experience.

Bryan Lask
Eating Disorders Research Team, St George's Hospital Medical School, London

Foreword

Cathy Malchiodi

Many years ago when I was a novice art therapist at a public high school in California, I stumbled upon a group of teenage girls in the lavatory vomiting. My naive impression was that they had contracted food poisoning from eating at the school cafeteria. When I asked if they needed my assistance or if they wanted to see the school nurse, one girl laughed and explained to me that they were not in fact ill. She pointed out to me that this was a good way 'to eat what you want and as much as you want and never gain weight'.

The girls I encountered that day were purposely purging themselves on a regular basis and were exhibiting what we now recognize today as bulimia. But at the time, my clinical supervisors could tell me very little about why these girls were purging and even less about what to do about it therapeutically. Literature and research studies on eating disorders such as bulimia and its counterpart, anorexia, were scarce; and nothing had been written on the use of creative art therapies to evaluate and treat these conditions.

Several years later a young woman was referred to my art therapy practice for emotional and physical problems that were interfering with her relationships and academic performance. To my surprise, she was one of the original group of girls that I had met in the high school lavatory purging themselves after a meal. The bulimia that began during her adolescence had continued into her young adulthood, and now its effects had not only impacted on emotional and interpersonal areas of her life, but had also taken their toll on her health and ability to complete her college degree. During our first session she expressed to me a sense of hopelessness about her body image and her inability to stop bingeing and purging no matter what she tried. She was also extremely depressed and addicted to laxatives and diuretics, which she used in an attempt to control her weight.

I think back to my encounter with that group of adolescents in the high school lavatory and my eventual meeting with this young woman, and I wish that I had had Susan Makin's book to guide me in my work with clients with eating disorders at that time. Makin has pulled together a rich variety of resources, information and ideas for intervention and treatment in what can often be difficult client cases. She has generously provided the reader with insights from her own vast experience with individuals with eating disorders and has thoughtfully prepared practical advice on individual and group approaches, materials and processes.

First and foremost this book conveys why art therapy is such a powerful and necessary modality in work with clients with eating disorders. Elise Warriner, explaining her personal experiences with an eating disorder, notes: 'Strange as it may seem, anorexia and illustration have at least one thing in common. They are both about expressing oneself without words, yet one is destructive and the other creative' (Warriner 1995, p.24). Ironically, eating disorders often turn out to be ways to numb pain, hide authentic expression and cover up depression, anxiety and fears. In contrast, art expression is a way to bring the internal pain out into the open and can become a way for those struggling with bulimia or anorexia to find hope, restoration and healing.

This book will greatly enhance your understanding of eating disorders and of why art therapy is an effective modality in treatment. Makin illustrates throughout this text that art therapy, in the hands of the skilled therapist or clinician, has the unique ability to make personal experiences tangible and to transform and repair mind, body and spirit. She provides the reader with skills, directions and insights that will help not only the beginner but also the advanced practitioner to apply creative media to their clinical work. Most importantly, Susan Makin is a caring and sensitive therapist whose extensive experience and timely advice make this book a valued resource for all clinicians working with this difficult, and often mysterious, population.

Cathy A. Malchiodi, ATR, LPAT, LPCC, REAT
Director, Institute for the Arts & Health, Salt Lake City, Utah

Reference

Warriner, E. (1995) 'Anger is red.' In D. Dokter (ed) *Arts Therapies and Clients with Eating Disorders: Fragile Board.* London: Jessica Kingsley Publishers.

Dedication

To all those with eating disorders who have found comfort, acceptance and hope in the art therapy process; and to the enlightened clinicians, administrators and teachers who have provided me with opportunities for professional and personal growth to enable me to amass and share the knowledge contained in this book.

Acknowledgements

Ellen Berlin; Ruth Chernia; Olinda Dimas; Lloyd Gilbert; Cindy Hardy; Peggy Osna Heller; Kathleen Kerr; Sharon Kirsch; Bryan Lask; Angela Lynde-Sinclair; Lev Makin; Shirley and Rex Makin; Cathy Malchiodi; George Mentis; Mary Neill; Gail Parsons; Steve Rojcewicz; Inderpal Salvja; Mark Sawyer; Gary Senter; Afsaneh Shafai; Joy Shuman; Shirley Sinclair; Eating Disorders Association (EDA); Eating Disorders Awareness and Prevention (EDAP); National Eating Disorder Information Centre (NEDIC); all the patients who so generously contributed their time, artwork, writing and input for this book; and Helen Parry and all those at Jessica Kingsley Publishers.

Testimony to art therapy

Art therapy has helped me express my feelings when I was too shy or self-conscious to show them. Through drawings and writing I've learned more about myself. Often I find hidden meanings in words I use, pictures I draw or sculpture I make.

I'm glad I have something to look back on, something to remind me of all the hard work I've done here and of the kindness that has been showered onto me. I am grateful for all the help I've received and I know I've accomplished a lot.

Perhaps now when I feel as though I cannot express my feelings, I will feel confident enough to sit down and write or draw a picture of my emotions. I don't run away from them any more, I face them, deal with them and move on.

Hopefully, I can do the same with my eating disorder, face it, deal with it and move on from it.

by someone recovering from an eating disorder

The magnitude of eating disorders

It is very hard to collect accurate statistics for eating disorders; different studies show different figures. This is, in part, because eating disorders tend to be secretive illnesses, and some of those affected are reluctant to admit to the problem (EDA 1999).

In the United States...

- Americans spend over $40 billion on dieting and diet-related products each year.
- Five to ten million girls and women and one million boys and men are struggling with eating disorders.
- Eighty per cent of American women are dissatisfied with their appearance.
- Forty-one per cent of 1st to 3rd graders want to be thinner.
- Eighty-one per cent of ten-year-olds are afraid of being fat.
- The average American woman is 5 ft 4 in tall and weighs 140 pounds. The average American model is 5 ft 11 in tall and weighs 117 pounds. Most fashion models are thinner than 98 per cent of American women.
- Thirty-five per cent of 'normal dieters' progress to pathological dieting. Of those, 20 to 25 per cent progress to partial or full syndrome eating disorders.
- Twenty-five per cent of American men and 45 per cent of American women are on a diet on any given day.

(According to EDAP 1999)

Introduction

What is a meal? In years gone by, a meal was often an occasion – a time for families, communities and guests to gather together and regale in others' company while sharing food. At a few festive times of the year, meals of this nature still happen. But, more often than not, in between, all kinds of anxieties build. Will Bill get on with Cathy? Should we invite Caroline? Is Claire trying to lose weight? Is Sheila on a wheat-free diet? Will Frank come and join us after the soccer game if he wins?

Not that earlier days were tension-free, but now as technology has become more sophisticated, so have our problems and avoidance techniques. Why do fast-food outlets outnumber restaurants that serve full-course meals? And, at the extreme, why are meal replacement bars the 'in' food of the new millennium?

In six barely-felt bites we can escape the time, effort, ritual and interaction that sharing a meal can involve. And for those who have no choice but to eat alone in our increasingly 'singles society', the pain of that can be brushed right under the carpet. A visit to the gym usually makes the evening complete.

Traditional accounts about the nature of eating disorders almost all discuss the mother–child relationship and early feeding experiences. However, even those form no particular pattern today. Relationships with mother as primary caregiver are not necessarily the norm, since single fathers and social support services assume nurturing responsibilities that used to be undertaken by mothers alone, and were taken for granted as such.

So what is happening to our society? And what is happening to our eating disorders? Why and how do they play themselves out? Is it because a meal is no longer a meal, or because we can no longer be who we think we are or who we are supposed to be or want to be? Of course, there is a lot more to eating disorders than just this, as will be shown here.

In exploring the treatment of eating disorders with art therapy, we cannot fail to make comparisons between art-making materials and food and how both are consumed. In regular verbal therapy, you have the therapist and the patient and the food and related eating and associated behaviours about which there is plenty of talk. However, only the patient and the therapist have voices. In art therapy, you have the therapist, the patient and the art product. All have their own voices. Meals are not just intangible contrived descriptions; they are actually represented by tangible spontaneously made art pieces.

The artwork, whether in the form of a sculpture or poem, in its own unique way offers background details that dialogue between therapist and patient may not. It is a representative of the patient's unconscious or newly conscious thoughts, feelings, and accounts. Not only does it take the stress – even the responsibility – away from the patient while the piece is being made (the 'enactment phase'), but also when it is viewed later (the 'observation/ reflection phase'). This is particularly important when the patient is not present, so that tendencies for 'mis-projections' (others ascribing meanings to a piece that its creator did not intend) do not happen.

Sometimes when looking at a piece, nothing needs to be said out loud by the patient, therapist, or other treatment team members. And then there are the times when the patient ends up saying a lot – a lot more than she could have said had she not made the piece and did not have it in front of her. At this point it cannot be emphasized enough that only the creator of an art piece can discuss what it might represent. The therapist may ask open-ended questions to prompt but cannot 'force-feed' or 'supplement' her offerings.

So, art therapy in the treatment of eating disorders is *more than just a meal*. Though it can help confirm all the expected and understandable issues that eating disordered patients have, it also goes much further. Through the process of play, meditation and expressive soul searching, art therapy is the indispensable kitchen hand that causes the master chef's creations to surpass the norm. In multidisciplinary approaches to treatment in particular, the greater the variety of complementary methodologies, the greater the chance of providing a five-star buffet in which every patient will be able to find something. Of all the disciplines offered for treatment, only art therapy has the ingredients to provide a multidimensional, sensual, and patient-centred approach simultaneously. Hence the title of this book: *More Than Just a Meal*.

The use of titles describing the order of a meal for the three parts of this book – Appetizers, The Main Course, Dessert – may seem corny, even offensive to some. Nevertheless, the decision to stay with them was encouraged by some patients recovering from their eating disorders. A meal is a metaphor for so much more, even the structure of a book. And once the 'meal plan' format was approved, the chapters seemed to come together and flow more naturally. Also, it is important to remember that humour has a very significant place in therapy, as will be seen in some of the examples of artwork in the second part of this book.

This book can be read from cover to cover, or chapters of particular interest can be read separately. The first part, 'Appetizers,' discusses the nature of eating disorders, who has them, what they are and how they are treated. There is then an overview of my approach to the arts therapies; my focus on association-making and use of media is pivotal, first, through the visual arts, and, second, through writing.

'The Main Course' looks at patterns that emerge as patients with eating disorders work with the arts therapies. The examples of patients' artwork, writing and reviews included here are from an arts therapies group held in an in-patient treatment programme. In addition to a series of miscellaneous art pieces and poems created by a variety of patients at different stages of treatment, three longer case excerpts focus on the efficacy of creative journalling.

'Dessert' looks at the road ahead. It considers where the reader, patient, parent, friend or therapist may want to go next after reading, and lists useful international and community resources. As well, my companion book, *Therapeutic Art Directives and Resources: Activities and Initiatives for Individuals and Groups* (Makin 1999), contains supplementary information for therapists. This includes lists of essential art-making supplies, suggestions for art-making directives in groups and for individuals, information on setting up a creative journal, and a creative journalling kit model. The conclusion considers the value of the arts therapies, particularly art therapy, as a treatment modality for eating disorders, both for self-help and in professional settings.

Throughout this book, I have chosen to refer to those engaged in art therapy as patients and have used the feminine *she* or *her* in describing them, as well as art(s) therapists. This is because most examples are taken from a hospital setting in which the majority (but not all) of the patients seen were women, as are most art(s) therapists. Also I often use the more inclusive term *arts therapies* (as opposed to *art therapy*) because, though my emphasis is on visual art-making, I do employ other arts modalities as well (particularly writing).

Michèle Wood (1996, p.18) talks about previous publications on eating disorders and art therapy:

> Most writers have chosen to describe their work in this area in terms of the clients' relationships with their families, particularly mothers, and with food, and their relationships with the art materials and the therapist. The effects of factors such as the institutional setting of the therapy, the person, body and gender of the therapist, and the effects of work done by other members of the multi-disciplinary team (where the art therapist is a member of such a team) have not been discussed.

Wood also notes that all art therapists who have consistently written in this area are women, and that it would be interesting to explore how gender issues within the therapeutic relationship might affect outcomes. I am mindful of these commentaries in my composition of this book and regret any limitations.

I would also like to mention here that this book is neither a handbook on eating disorders or the arts therapies, nor a critique of treatment approaches or healthcare systems. I invite you to approach the book with an open mind and heart and discover the art of eating disorders and everything that they represent and is attached to them.

PART I

Appetizers

It is more than time for the great many of us who work experientially with patients who suffer from eating disorders to begin to build a body of literature that supports the efficacy of our work.

(Alpers 1997, p.105)

CHAPTER I

Introducing Eating Disorders

This introduction offers an overview of information about eating disorders that focuses on anorexia nervosa and bulimia nervosa. In considering their history, incidence, natures, treatments and medications, as well as advice for those who are close to people with eating disorders, the emphasis is on prevalent trends in modern Western society, particularly in North America and Britain.

1. History

Eating disorders have been evident for hundreds of years. In England, Richard Morton first wrote about 'nervous consumption' in 1689. In England and France in the mid-1800s, there was an increased interest in this problem, leading to Sir William Gull coining the term 'anorexia nervosa' in 1868 and defining a clear symptomatology.

In the late 1800s, anorexia nervosa was viewed as a 'pure' psychiatric disorder. However, this was reversed at the turn of the century as physicians attached more importance to the presenting physical emaciation; the term 'anorexia nervosa' fell into disuse. Only in the late 1930s was anorexia nervosa re-established as a disease of psychological origin. Even so, approaches to treatment remain divided according to emphasis on the physiological or psychological problems.

According to Batal *et al.* (1998), bulimia was only defined in English literature as a separate clinical entity by Russell in 1979. (However, bingeing and purging dates back to the aristocracy of ancient Rome, who purged in their 'vomitoriums' as a matter of common practice.) The first conference on eating disorders took place in 1984, and *The International Journal of Eating Disorders* was established at that time.

2. Incidence

The causes of eating disorders are manifold. However, it is generally believed that problems arise because of a psychological disturbance involving feelings of poor self-esteem, helplessness and ineffectiveness. It is also interesting to note that there is a higher rate of eating disorders among the children of parents with such disorders, which suggests that some of the tendencies may have been learned by example or that there could be genetic reasons. In the same way, siblings also have a greater propensity towards the disorder.

Anorexia nervosa is most prevalent in industrialized societies, where food is plentiful and popular culture places a high value on slimness. In the United States, it is said to affect approximately 1 per cent of women, traditionally starting in adolescence and peaking at ages 14 and 18 (Mehler, Gray and Schulte 1997). Again, in the United States, bulimia nervosa is said to affect approximately 1 to 2 per cent of the entire population (Batal *et al.* 1998); very frequently, those affected show some aspects of the two illnesses.

According to the EDA's (1997) Statistics regarding eating disorders, in Britain, about 60,000 people may have anorexia nervosa or bulimia nervosa at any one time, and 8.1 new cases of anorexia nervosa and 11.4 cases of bulimia nervosa are recorded per 100,000 population annually. Also in the 10 to 19 age range, family doctors identify 34.1 cases of anorexia nervosa and 41 cases of bulimia nervosa per 100,000 population each year. And in the 20 to 39 age range, the number of cases of bulimia nervosa rises to 56.7.

Males with eating disorders generally account for 5 to 10 per cent of anorexia nervosa cases (Mehler *et al.* 1997) and 10 per cent of bulimia nervosa cases. It is estimated that among school-age children, as many as 25 per cent of those with eating disorders may be male (EDA 1997). According to Arnold Anderson (1998), men often start starving themselves to change their body shape (usually their abdomen): 'Men are dissatisfied from the waist up, and women, from the waist down.' The figure for high school and college-age students who will manifest bulimic symptoms at some time during their studies is at 15 per cent (Batal *et al.* 1998).

Although identified cases of eating disorders are on the rise, it is questioned whether this is due to a greater incidence or to a greater recognition of the illness by doctors. And, unfortunately, neither anorexia nervosa nor bulimia nervosa tends to be transitory. Without treatment, they can continue for decades, significantly impairing all aspects of life from work and health to relationships with others, if they do not kill the sufferer first.

Discussing eating disorders in Hong Kong, Sing Lee (1998) asks that we not consider eating disorders as being non-existent in non-Western societies. It is just that Western research materials may not be applicable in these cultures. And Janet Treasure (1998), quoting Palm's research, reminds us that of the 5,000,000 people in the world with anorexia nervosa 4,999,999 were not in clinical trials.

Marsha Marcus (1998), President of the Academy for Eating Disorders (a US research organization with a selective, nominated membership of 500), also points out that 40 per cent of women are trying to lose weight at any given time: 'Food and food-related behaviour has become a marker of moral inferiority and superiority in our culture ... you are what you eat.' And according to Stein *et al.* (1998), 15 to 45 per cent of people with partial eating disorders will develop full eating disorders after a couple of years.

Estimations of mortality rates vary, but as many as 10 to 15 per cent of sufferers of eating disorders die from related complications. In fact, the morbidity and mortality rates for anorexia nervosa are probably the highest recorded for any psychiatric disorder and are on the rise. Anorexia nervosa is the third most chronic illness among teenage girls (EDA 1997). Anorexics die from the many secondary effects of prolonged starvation; bulimics, from having deranged their metabolic systems, depleting their bodies of potassium, and causing abnormal heart rhythms and cardiac arrest. Sufferers of both of these diseases also have a higher risk of suicide.

3. Anorexia nervosa

According to John M. Cleghorn and Betty Lou Lee, 'thin is in' in modern Western society (Cleghorn and Lee 1991, p.137). Anorexics are described as people who are unusually obsessed with food, but cannot bring themselves to eat it. In the pursuit of thinness, many of them literally starve themselves to death, while insisting that they are still too fat; it is not that they have no appetite or are uninterested in food.

At first, limiting food intake generally gives anorexics a sense of being in control, but does nothing to resolve the (real) underlying problems. In many cases, they have to continue to diet to feel in control and this leads to either starvation or food binges (with the subsequent purges). A vicious cycle is established. The emotional effects of their eating/not eating patterns bring about irritability, depressed mood and poor concentration. Hence, their original psychological and physical problems are also exacerbated, increasing their drive to further dieting.

The DSM-IV (*Diagnostic and Statistical Manual of Mental Disorders*, fourth edition) defines anorexia nervosa as involving the following criteria (American Psychiatric Association 1994):

1. A refusal to maintain body weight at or above a minimally normal weight for age and height (less than 85% of that expected).

2. An intense fear of gaining weight and becoming fat, even though underweight.

3. An undue influence of body shape or weight on self-image, or denial of the seriousness of the current low body weight.

4. Amenorrhoea: the missing of three consecutive menstrual periods.

There are also two types of anorexia nervosa: restricting and binge eating/purging. However, as American eating disorders researcher Timothy Walsh (1995) points out, there is sometimes no 'hard and fast line' in distinguishing overdieting from anorexia nervosa.

The medical complications of anorexia nervosa usually result from starvation; cardiac problems are the most common cause of sudden death. An overview of the main physiological systems, and complications arising in them, follows.

Cardiovascular

Anorexics can demonstrate extreme fatigue that is usually linked to hypotension (very low blood pressure). However, according to Mehler *et al.* (1997), once an anorexic's electrocardiograph is found to be normal, routine screening is not necessary. They point out that the period of greatest risk for clinical cardiac decompensation is not at the lowest point of weight loss, but during the first two weeks of refeeding.

'Refeeding syndrome' was first evident in World War II concentration camp survivors, who died after being refed with high carbohydrate food. Similarly for anorexics, calorific nutrients, especially those high in glucose, whether taken in through eating or intravenously, can cause cardiovascular collapse and death.

Endocrine

The most obvious endocrine complication is amenorrhoea (cessation of menstrual periods), which is now one of the diagnostic criteria for anorexia nervosa. And according to Mehler *et al.* (1997), the carrying on of anorexic behaviours, together with emotional stress, once weight has been regained, often does not allow for the resumption of normal menses.

Mehler *et al.* also explain that the amenorrhoea associated with anorexics is not only related to weight loss, since it happens prior to significant weight loss in as many as 50 per cent of patients, and continues despite eating becoming more normal and weight being regained. Pointing to studies on anorexics' recovery of their periods, they note that the rates of persistent amenorrhoea can range from 5 per cent to 44 per cent.

Another significant endocrine complication of anorexia nervosa as explained by Mehler *et al.* is severe osteoporosis, which is irreversible. This condition is regarded as extremely serious because the usually early age of onset of the illness is at the time when maximum skeletal growth and mineralization normally occur. Thus, there is much concern about long-term health consequences.

Gastrointestinal

Anorexics have less severe gastrointestinal problems than bulimics. However, there are serious disturbances involving bloating and constipation.

Central nervous

Cerebral atrophy and brain volume shrinkage are the most obvious complications of the central nervous system. However, according to Mehler *et al.* (1997), normal brain volumes are restored in nearly all patients who recover from anorexia nervosa. And generalized muscle weakness, anorexics' most common neurological complaint, also dissipates with recovery.

Dermatological

Dermatological complications include dry scaly skin, brittle nails and hair, and the growth of lanugo-like body hair on arms, legs, the back and face (for the conservation of body heat). All are completely reversible with weight gain.

Mehler *et al.* (1997) record the aggregate annual mortality rate associated with anorexia nervosa as being 12 times higher than the annual death rate in the general population, for all causes of death for women 15 to 24 years old. Thus, no more than 50 per cent of anorexic patients make a complete recovery.

4. Bulimia nervosa

According to Cleghorn and Lee (1991), people with bulimia nervosa, like anorexics, are said to have a morbid fear of fatness. However, they are not readily spotted by their size. Since they binge and purge (by frequent self-induced vomiting, obsessive exercising and laxative misuse), they can be under, over or normal weight. With periodic feeding frenzies, as many as 6000 calories can be gobbled down by bulimics in an hour, usually in secret.

Bulimia has been described as a 'growth industry', both commercially and in incidence in recent years. 'Bulimia nervosa' describes the 'full-blown' syndrome, while 'bulimia' refers to the purging alone.

The DSM-IV defines bulimia nervosa as involving the following criteria:

1. Recurrent episodes of binge eating, which involves eating in a discrete period of time a larger amount of food than most people would during a similar period under similar conditions, and a sense of lack of control over that eating.

2. Recurrent, inappropriate compensatory behaviours to prevent weight gain, such as self-induced vomiting and misuse of laxatives, diuretics and diet pills, occurring more than twice a week.

3. The binge eating and inappropriate compensatory behaviours each occur at least twice a week over a three-month period.

4. An overconcern with weight and body shape, affecting self-image.

5. The disturbance does not only occur during episodes of anorexia nervosa.

There are, also, two types of bulimia nervosa – purging and non-purging.

Bulimia nervosa is more common than anorexia nervosa. But, as already mentioned, it is less obvious because the bulimic does not necessarily have a low body weight. Nevertheless, there are a number of behaviours specific to bulimia nervosa, which centre around secrecy and shame and therefore provide their own special challenges. And although the prognosis is better than for anorexia nervosa, medical complications related to purging do arise.

Batal *et al.* (1998) list certain physical manifestations that may well be indicators of bulimia nervosa. These include enlarged salivary glands (from vomiting), abrasions from teeth to the upper surface of the hand (from inducing vomiting), extensive dental problems (especially erosions), severe inflammation of the oesophagus, recurrent low levels of potassium and acid-base imbalance. In general, as Batal *et al.* discuss, medical complications of bulimia relate to modes of purging. An overview of the main purging modes, and complications arising from them, follows.

Self-induced vomiting

Complications arising from self-induced vomiting involve the oral cavity and oesophagus. This is due to the constant regurgitation of acidic gastric contents. Thus, common dental complications are perimyolysis (the wearing away of the enamel on the surface of the front teeth close to the tongue) and gingivitis (gum disease). According to Batal *et al.*, enamel erosion is a common manifestation in 38 per cent of bulimic patients. They also note that visible enamel destruction usually happens after about two years of regular vomiting episodes.

Hypertrophy of the salivary glands and swelling at the back of the neck are other complications arising from vomiting, which, according to Batal *et al.*, occur in 10 to 50 per cent of bulimic patients. This swelling is usually painless, bilateral and quite noticeable, and its frequency and severity are directly proportional to the frequency of the vomiting.

Also, according to Batal *et al.*, up to 50 per cent of bulimic patients who are self-induced vomiters often have gastrointestinal problems such as heartburn, dysphagia (the act of swallowing being hard or painful) and odynophagia (a burning sensation or pain being felt after swallowing). It is also important to consider the serious losses of electrolytes (sodium and potassium).

While most self-induced vomiting is by means of the insertion of a finger or utensil into the throat, some turn to ipecac (a substance usually used to help eliminate acute overdoses of household toxins). When ipecac is abused, severe poisoning can be caused; most of this toxicity is to skeletal muscle and the heart, involving tachycardia (higher than normal heart rate), dyspnoea (laboured or difficult breathing), hypotension (abnormally low blood pressure) and arrhythmias (irregular heartbeats).

Laxative abuse

According to Batal *et al.*, the relative risk among bulimic patients for incidence of laxative abuse is 3.5 times that of the general population. However, it should be noted that laxatives cannot influence weight control, since they work on the large intestine after calories have already been absorbed in the small intestine. There are five major types of laxatives, and the ones most abused by bulimic patients are the 'stimulants'. These include compounds containing pheolphthalein and anthraquinone, which act quickly to induce bowel movements in which significant amounts of watery diarrhoea are produced.

Medical complications of laxative abuse have effects on both the gastro-intestinal system and electrolytes (chloride, calcium, bicarbonate and potassium). Also, it should be noted that laxative withdrawal is not an easy process, because of rebound constipation and fluid retention, not to forget the anxieties attached to feeling out of control.

Diuretic abuse

Like laxatives, diuretics (drugs that increase the volume of urine produced by promoting the excretion of salts and water from the kidney) are unsuccessful at facilitating weight loss. And temporary losses of two to four pounds from dehydration are usually followed by fluid retention and weight gain. As with laxatives, the major complications of their abuse involve electrolyte abnorm-alities that can lead to heart arrhythmias. There can also be manifestations of nausea, constipation and abdominal pain. Diuretics are less frequently abused by bulimic patients than are laxatives.

Diet pills

Batal *et al.* comment that diet pills, despite being one of the most effective ways of controlling weight, as a possible mode of purging, are seldom used by bulimia patients because of their side-effects. These include palpitations, anxiety attacks, headaches, elevated blood pressure and seizures.

Case reports on the coexistence of bulimia and type 1 diabetes (insulin-dependent diabetes mellitus) started to appear in the early 1930s. Batal *et al.* note that the incidence of type 1 diabetes is 10 to 15 per 100,000 people per year in North America, occurring mostly in children and adolescents. And from 1 to 3 per cent of adolescent girls and young women in North America are bulimic.

Batal *et al.* also discuss the controversial question of whether there is increased incidence of bulimia among young women with type 1 diabetes or merely an overlap of two common illnesses. They cite multiple studies that show 30 to 50 per cent of young women with type 1 diabetes practise disordered eating behaviours to control their weight. In fact, up to 50 per cent of diabetic women have been reported as being binge eaters.

Another common practice of diabetic women is to reduce or omit insulin doses to induce weight loss by means of osmotic diuresis with glycosuria (increased urination involving the elimination of abnormally high amounts of glucose). The name given to this behaviour is 'insulin purging'.

Fewer outcome data are available for anorexia nervosa than bulimia nervosa. But in general, according to Batal *et al.*, more than 80 per cent of patients are expected to have a 'meaningful recovery', and negative outcomes are usually found in those who are substance abusers or who have a lower body weight.

5. Treatments and medications

Treatments and medications for eating disorders are subjects of much discussion in academic literature and quantitative research analyses. However, despite all the discussion and research, eating disorders remain fatal illnesses, with many sufferers having poor responses to both treatment and medication. This is curious, despite the increasing number of highly trained specialists in the field.

Melanie Katzman (1998), a much respected eating disorders specialist, speaking at the Eighth New York International Conference on Eating Disorders, made these interesting remarks: 'Who is obsessed by "fat", the patients or observers/practitioners?' 'Today's specialists know a lot about a little!' 'If eating disorders are the answer, what is the problem?'

Treatments

Treatments for eating disorders are usually of two types. First, there are medical treatments that give attention to any physical damage done while establishing new eating patterns. Second, there are medical and psycho-therapeutic treatments that help deal with the problems (psychological or physical, or both) that activated the whole cycle in the beginning.

In out-patient care, the first phase of treatment usually involves the formation of a 'contract' concerning the maintenance of a certain weight in order to avoid hospitalization. Admission to a hospital for periods of up to several months is advisable for those patients who need intensive monitoring of their food intake and nutritional status and who are physically at risk, with 'normal' eating patterns being set during this time.

In a few cases, feeding through intravenous or naso-gastric tubes may even be required. Long-term, ongoing aftercare is recommended to help solve many of the resulting and precipitating family, interpersonal and social issues generated.

Medications

Some researchers claim that antidepressants can bring about dramatic results with bulimics. Also, contemporary findings in brain chemistry and the systems that regulate feeding are pointing to new agents which may be useful. However, much more research on them is imperative, so that safety and effectiveness are proved over extended periods of time. Research indicates that one reason for bulimia may be a low level of serotonin, 'a chemical in the brain that sends out signals like: 'That's enough. You're full' (Cleghorn and Lee 1991, p.141).

Irrespective of treatments and medications used, researchers have found that 95 to 98 per cent of regular dieters not only regain all the weight they lost, but gain even more. It is thought that this is due to the human body having a 'set point' weight range which it naturally settles at. There is little a person can do about her set point because it is genetic.

Also, the body is not able to tell the difference between voluntary dieting and imposed famine, and thus it will do everything possible to protect and maintain itself. Consequently, it will lower its metabolic rate (the rate at which calories are burned) to keep its set point. It is noted that over a five-year period most people regain all the weight they have lost and more, and their set point is raised accordingly to protect itself in case there be another imposed famine period.

6. Advice for family, friends and co-workers

According to Mehler *et al.* (1997), certain occupational groups are more at risk for anorexia nervosa than others. These include actors, singers, dancers, athletes, skaters, models, wrestlers, gymnasts, jockeys, flight attendants, students (school, college and university) and others for whom thinness is considered to be an asset.

It is important to be aware of those who are close to us and whether they are crying out for help, silently and not so silently. And if they are, how and when to intervene is a delicate matter requiring patience, time and diplomacy. Here are a number of recommendations, adapted from the National Eating Disorder Information Centre's 'Guide for Family and Friends of a Person Experiencing Food and Weight Problems'. They may be helpful, depending on the situation.

1. *Do not force someone with an eating disorder to get help*
    Although it can be extremely frustrating, we cannot seek help for a person with an eating disorder; only they can choose to do so, of the kind that they need, and when they are ready.

2. *Let the person with an eating disorder identify her own issues, when she is ready, choosing appropriate treatment sources*
    Eating disorders happen for many reasons, but deeper problems that are too difficult and painful to address directly are at the root of most of them. So, there are many layers to eating disorders for those suffering from them to come to terms with and for which to seek help. It is important for the sufferer to be able to identify what is really bothering her, so that she can seek help that will work for her.

3. *Wait to be approached by the person with the eating disorder*
    People with eating disorders seldom welcome others' expressions of concern and often react with anger and denial. They are usually only ready to talk when they know that those around them are concerned but are not going to impose treatments on them before they are ready.

4. *Avoid commenting on appearances*
    It is very hard and unnatural not to give comments about weight and looks, especially if you feel that they will be complimentary. Since people with eating disorders are overly focused on these already, comments will only perpetuate their body image obsessions.

5. *Avoid power struggles around food and eating*
    Eating disorders often revolve around needs for control. So, being able to be in charge of what, how and when one eats can be a replacement for lack of control felt in other areas of life.

Consequently, the forcing and tempting of people with eating disorders to eat may only aggravate disordered eating patterns.

6. *An individual can only go at her own pace for getting better*
    Leaving the door open for discussion can make it feel easier and safer for people with eating disorders to consider getting help sooner. Sensitivity in offering appropriate information at appropriate times is extremely difficult but important for allowing those with eating disorders to see alternatives to the present situation. Also, staying in treatment settings that do not meet their needs may further retard healing. It should be remembered that it sometimes takes years to start dealing with an eating disorder.

7. *Examine your own attitudes about body image and size*
    Often, we are not aware of how and when we might convey 'fat prejudice', enhancing the desire for thinness. Rather than telling someone with an eating disorder not to worry because they will never get fat, you might ask them to start looking at their fears about being fat and what they feel they can achieve by being thin. This may lead to the question: 'Is food restriction making you happier and helping you to achieve what you want, or is it creating more problems for you?' If you feel comfortable, it may be good to share ways you, personally, are affected by social pressures to be thin. Appropriate and timely sharing can help alleviate shame and discomfort for the other person.

8. *Be careful not to blame*
    It is often hard to keep our own anger and frustrations in check. If you are able to keep in mind that eating disorders are coping strategies for dealing with painful emotions and experiences, you will be less likely to blame people with eating disorders for their struggle.

9. *Do not take on the role of therapist*
    Although a therapist has been described as a good friend, there is a fine line. It is often beneficial for those close to someone with an eating disorder to seek some support themselves if they feel the need, so that they can be there appropriately for the other person, and in a way that is not harmful to either party.

10. *Remember that professionals in the field of eating disorders have their own limitations*

It is important to keep in mind that specialists in the field of eating disorders are human too. They make mistakes and have their own areas of weakness. Thus, who is administering treatment and the faith you have in them is significant. Also, more often than not, eating disorders professionals work in institutions or are subject to government healthcare legislation. Unfortunately, politics does not always put the patient first, and certain individuals, though worthy clinicians, do not always practise as is desirable because of external pressures placed on them by systems and other players in them.

This final point is a recommendation that I add from my own experiences and observations and, for me, is one of the most difficult and important to recognize and share.

CHAPTER 2

Introducing Art Therapy

I came to art therapy by a long and winding road. As a child, art-making was a natural instinct. And fortunately, my art-making inclinations were encouraged by my parents. So, when I moved away from the family home and came to face the perils of the wider world by myself, I had a familiar, approved comforter at hand. Art-making could be called upon at all times and for all reasons. Art-making helped me through loneliness, relocation, abuse, self-esteem issues and serious illness. With a paint brush or ballpoint pen, I consciously and unconsciously tackled current problems, old woes and future concerns in playful and meditative ways. Not only was this soothing, but my feelings about certain circumstances seemed to become clearer.

One spring, I decided to share my self-discovered comforter with others in a vacation job, a series of workshops that I named 'Art F.I.T.' (Art for Fun, Interest and Therapy). I thought that I had invented art therapy, then discovered that I had not. So, I went back to school to study the following: art therapy, expressive therapies and poetry therapy. My art therapy training and practical experiences led me to an in-patient eating disorders programme. There had not been an art therapist on the unit before, and I wasn't one when I started. Since then, nearly eight years have passed, and my skills have developed both as an art(s) therapist and eating disorders practitioner.

It is now time to share findings and techniques with other clinicians and the general public, and to discuss the important contribution of the arts therapies, particularly those involving visual arts and poetry, in the treatment of eating disorders. There were not many references to turn to on the subject when I began, and I learned much by trial and error.

1. The healing power of art

Sir Winston Churchill's eloquent description of the art-making process emphasizes the healing powers of art:

> Painting is complete as a distraction. I know of nothing which, without exhausting the body, more entirely absorbs the mind. Whatever the worries of the hour or the threats of the future, once the picture has begun to flow along, there is no room for them in the mental screen. They pass out into shadow and darkness. All one's mental light, such as it is, becomes concentrated on the task. Time stands respectfully aside. (1950, quoted in Edwards 1979, p.154)

Due to the powerful way that art can communicate feelings, artists in Western cultures have been both admired and ostracized for the impact that their art has had on its viewers. However, shamans from Eastern cultures have used art of many types in their healing rituals for centuries.

2. Art therapy historically

In western Europe, an interest in the art of the mentally ill started in France in the later 1800s. In 1872, psychiatrist Ambroise-Auguste Tardieu's *Études Medico-Légales sur la Folie* (Medico-Legal Studies of Madness) were written to establish objective criteria for a legally acceptable diagnosis of insanity. However, in North America, it was not until the 1940s that Margaret Naumburg and Edith Kramer started applying psychoanalytic theory to their work in art education and therapy with children. Naumburg combined art-making with verbal therapy, while Kramer viewed the process of art-making itself as therapy. Initially, North American art therapy developed from these two pioneers' leads.

3. Art therapy today

Internationally, art therapy is approached from many philosophical perspectives, and is used with individuals and groups in a variety of settings. The British Art Therapy Association now numbers approximately 1300 members, including about 1000 who are state registered and 80 students. The American Art Therapy Association now numbers approximately 3625, with 2110 registered members and 417 student members.

The contemporary American expressive arts therapist and educator Shaun McNiff described his particular approach to art therapy in his first book, *The Arts and Psychotherapy* (1981):

Through expressive art therapy the client is given the opportunity to renew the artistic consciousness within a trusting environment that responds directly to idiosyncratic needs and expressive problems. Each person is encouraged to rediscover his personal expressive style. Artistic techniques and methods are introduced only to the extent that they support the person's expression and further creative discovery. (p.48)

There is an increasing trend to merge art therapy with the other arts therapies; the new International Expressive Arts Therapy Association (IEATA), with a mostly North American membership, numbers 460, with 320 professional members and 140 student members. It includes art therapists, those combining art therapy with other disciplines (arts and otherwise), and other arts therapies practitioners such as movement, music and poetry therapists.

4. Art therapy's advantages

Art therapy can be beneficial for a whole range of human conditions. Neurotic, psychotic, physically impaired, hyperactive, inhibited or 'normal' individuals of all ages and in all states can have positive experiences using it. Our inner urges to express not only conscious but unconscious or repressed thoughts and feelings are given a lot of freedom in the art room setting, where spontaneity is encouraged. However, at first it can be difficult to be spontaneous, because of our tendency to screen and control our actions that becomes second nature with age.

Concrete evidence of individuals' internal changes is shown when the style, contents and techniques of the art-making experience are reviewed and discussed with an arts therapist, who acts as witness and guide. Challenges in art-making usually reflect those confronted in life. So, when pictures or sculptures that may not be 'pretty' are able to be made, communications become more direct and honest. And with less need to create aesthetically beautiful pieces of artwork, the overall experience can be more therapeutic and healing. Different aspects of what someone may be going through are displayed, both during the art-making process and through the artwork created. Therefore, as information comes up and is recognized, the development of problem-solving abilities and emotional maturation are prompted and supported. When a series of paintings or sculptures is reviewed and discussed, the individual who has created them is helped to see how patterns can emerge and that symbolic messages are understood. So, the art therapy experience over time and as a whole (art-making, artwork, review and discussion) becomes ego-supportive, promoting a healthier sense of identity.

Language, a principal means of communication, can strongly inhibit some individuals' freedom to be emotionally expressive (the verbally withdrawn, verbose, foreign language speaking, or auditorily and speech impaired). Art therapy, however, provides all with an opportunity to express unconscious or hard-to-communicate thoughts and feelings by projecting them visually or symbolically. Also, in group art therapy, people from different backgrounds (ethnic, racial, social, economic, educational, and so on) are able to come together with relative ease, making use of art as a universal mode of communication. Dr Martin Fischer, founder of the Toronto Art Therapy Institute, (1913–1992) often used to say that the symbolism expressed in spontaneous art-making emphasizes 'the universality of the inner reality of man'.

Artwork produced in art therapy is valuable for diagnosis as well as for therapy, because certain signs and symbols are easily identifiable. People suffering from particular conditions usually create pictures and sculptures that reflect their conditions. So, looking at a series of artworks made by an individual over a period of time can reveal a better understanding of his or her condition and any changes in it. Also, developmental psychologists researching the primacy of childhood images have found that experiences belonging to the pre-verbal realm of infancy cannot be adequately expressed in words. Art therapy provides the opportunity to bring these experiences to the surface with visual symbolism.

5. The art therapy process

During the art-making process, various materials are used that may facilitate the expression of repressed or conflicting thoughts and feelings. Trauma, fantasies, self-image questions, relationship concerns and impulse control issues are all projected in the artwork's imagery. This gives its creators stimuli for association-making. For me, association-making and the insights that are triggered by it hold one of the main keys to art therapy's power.

Patterns that emerge in an individual's artwork can be directly related to that person's life experiences and responses to them. An individual's psychological profile manifests itself progressively through the style and content of the artwork created, as well as the colours used in it. Colours have personal as well as universal meanings. These are usually given spontaneously and unconsciously. As well as expressing moods, how colours are applied can reveal ambivalent feelings and significant identifications with people, places and circumstances. Changes of colour, like changes in symbolism and subject matter, can show negative or positive developments on an individual's road to recovery.

Arts therapies processes enable individuals to overcome obstacles to self-expression in ways that other treatment methods cannot. This points out the significant gaps in psychotherapies that rely more exclusively on verbal communications.

6. Group art therapy

Group art therapy tends to be the preferred mode of treatment in in-patient settings, since it can work on several levels at the same time. Group members find non-verbal as well as verbal ways to communicate to others while being able to participate simultaneously, and at their own pace, in their own art-making. Thereby, individuals experience relative freedom from failure, or disharmony with other group members. And no matter how aggressive or uninhibited artwork might appear to be on the page, in reality it is not a danger to its creator or other group members.

Positive communications and congenial relationships tend to be fostered between group members in the art-making environment. These are often helpful in leading to the verbalization of strong emotions and sharing of experiences that might not happen in other settings.

7. Individual art therapy

In individual art therapy, the patient engaging in direct interaction with art materials makes a number of significant discoveries: alternative choices are possible, decisions have direct results, mistakes can be learned from, and fresh attempts can be made. The patient working alone in a personal creative journal is also able to make similar discoveries.

8. The art therapist's role

The art therapist acts as guide and witness, and is concerned with creating an environment in which the patient feels free and safe to create and communicate. The patient's active and voluntary association-making is essential for the art therapist to develop a more adequate understanding of a patient. After the patient has created a piece of artwork, the art therapist provides her with an opportunity to comment on its meaning and to talk about her associated thoughts and feelings. At this time, the patient has the opportunity to stress what is really important to her. Spontaneously created art and association-making not only reveal attitudes and conflicts, but also give information about an individual's intellectual capacity.

The art therapist can help stimulate free association-making by asking pertinent, but open, questions, such as: 'Does the artwork have a name? How do you feel about the colours that you have used in it? What do they mean to you? What mood do they reflect? Do you or don't you like the finished piece?' It is important, however, that the patient discover the meaning of her colours, designs and symbols for herself, and contribute actively and productively to her own growth, autonomy and objectivity. The art therapist not only guides and witnesses the patient during the art-making and verbal processing of the artwork, but also keeps records of the visual language produced for other team members to review at meetings, making sure that all associations to it are recorded in the patient's own words.

9. Susan's arts therapies approach

As I mentioned in the introduction to this book, adopting a profession in the arts therapies was a natural consequence for me. Art therapy was something that I had done spontaneously for myself since childhood; later on, it became something I was trained to practise with others. Now, after a number of years of practice, my methodology takes new twists, and I follow my own initiatives more confidently. I am more heavily engaged in intermodal work; that is, moving between the arts from art to writing, poem-making and reading, and back.

The outline given in this chapter relays the essentials of 'pure' art therapy. Some of the examples of patients' work in Part II of this book, however, reveal later 'trimmings' which focus on poetry writing and storytelling techniques. I have found that more detailed association-making (putting words to our art and art to our words) enhances the whole treatment process. And eating-disordered patients are particularly adept at moving and motivated to move between the media offered, ultimately evolving to find the technique of their personal 'comfort zone', and even enjoyment.

It is also important to keep in mind Wood's reminder: 'Techniques may well be determined by the clinical setting as well as the particular needs of any individual client' (Wood 1996, p.17). Though I had many ideas about what I wanted to do in the in-patient eating disorders setting in which I worked, I was invariably unable to go ahead with them, and had to work around the system employing me.

CHAPTER 3

Art Therapy and Eating Disorders

Although much has been written by arts therapists and others about the arts therapies, there has been little discussion of the application of art and poetry therapy with eating-disordered patients. Also, the majority of publications that do exist are divided between British and American authors. Most of the books tend to have British authorship and focus on specific theoretical orientations. Most of the articles tend to have American authorship, recounting personal experiences in their practices. I have found that substantial demonstrations of practical interventions that have universal application, particularly for new practitioners, are missing from the literature. I hope to remedy this, both in this book and its companion, *Therapeutic Art Directives and Resources: Activities and Initiatives for Individuals and Groups* (Makin 1999).

My own arts therapies practice emerged not only from the training programmes that I attended in the US and Canada, but also from knowledge sources such as conferences, professional associations, reading, and learning experiences on the job. And, beyond all of these, I am not afraid to acknowledge my own opinions, limitations and comfort zones.

My eclectic way of working crystallized over seven years spent in an in-patient eating disorders setting. Creating an arts therapies programme at a traditional Canadian teaching hospital was not without challenge. Time restrictions and budget constraints, coupled with team accountability, responsibilities and dynamics, were often very isolating. And being the only arts therapist in a large conservative hospital at a time of crisis in government healthcare policies caused me to be cautious.

I describe my methodology as a 'hybrid' way of working: a fairly directive and conservative approach within spontaneous parameters. That is, most of my sessions appeared fairly directed and structured; but beyond the initial instructions given at strategic points in them, and despite space and materials restrictions, patients were encouraged to be as spontaneous and creative as possible. Although this may appear somewhat contradictory, it is not:

patients and therapist ended up with the best of both worlds. Dr Martin Fischer, an early art therapy teacher of mine, used to say: 'You have to lose control to gain mastery.' My sessions accommodated this premise: though control was allowed to be lost, there were always points of focus to return to for grounding and safety.

As already mentioned, a significant amount of written material about eating disorders and art therapy is British. Michèle Wood, a British art therapist, gives a comprehensive overview of the British publications. Like Holly Matto, an American social worker, Wood notices that psychodynamic approaches are emphasized. The focus of treatment is not on the removal of the eating behaviour, but on understanding what it means and how patients are affected by it (on both sides of the Atlantic): 'Art-making is seen as providing the client with an alternative reality and the tools for creating something that may enable them to relinquish their self-destructive behaviour' (Wood 1996, p.13).

The remainder of this chapter considers, systematically and chronologically, other authors' descriptions of art therapy and eating-disordered patients' responses to it.

1. Art-making materials and eating disorders

When art-making materials are displayed on a table, participants are free to choose those that appeal to them. At a meal, the intention is to satisfy appetites for food; at an art-making session, expressive desires. The two settings are intimately related forums for satisfying unconscious needs. There is a lot of scope for comparison between the art-making materials we pick and how we use them, and why and how we select and eat our food. At one end of the continuum, anorexics tend to prefer to make faint crayon marks and work in very small dimensions. At the other end, bulimics can be very wasteful with art supplies. In the extreme, they pour paint over the page so thickly that it is often too sticky to dry, making a terrible mess on the surrounding work area. Anorexics show a desire to disappear from the page; bulimics make bold strokes all over the page and beyond.

Three art therapists in particular have discussed art-making materials in the context of their work with eating-disordered patients – Mari Fleming, Joy Schaverien and Holly Matto.

Mari Fleming

Mari Fleming, an American art therapist, focuses on art materials that are suitable for anorexic patients. At the initial stages of art therapy treatment, she recommends familiar and non-threatening media, such as pencils, markers and crayons, which are reassuring and calming. She also notes that these media usually encourage cognitive responses. Since intellectual abilities are a strength of many anorexics, cognitive responses that feel familiar and certain are a helpful stimulus. For the anorexic who is apprehensive, however, the direction to make a collage or place a border around the paper may provide additional encouragement (Fleming 1989).

At a mid-stage of art therapy treatment, Fleming encourages expression of affect and self-investigation. This, she recommends, can be achieved with media such as soft pastels, oil pastels and paint. However, she warns that thick paint may encourage regression, due to its smearing and running capacities and to its similarity to body fluids. Alternatively, she notes how clay both invites regression (because of its similar 'goopy' qualities) and supports reintegration (because of its capacity for cohesion). One tip for when patients experience anxiety, Fleming notes, is to return to materials that they have previously experienced as safe or soothing.

Fleming explains how the focus at the termination stage of art therapy treatment should be on issues of loss and possible regression to early needs. So, she advocates that previous artwork and experiences be reconsidered to facilitate exploration of anxiety, rage and guilt. Thus, self-understanding, a cohesive sense of self, and constructive defences can be supported. At this time, she recommends returning to the art media used at the initial stages of treatment for soothing and to help with closure. Fleming states: 'Control over the art material provides a substitute, or outlet, for wishes of control previously manifested in eating behavior and preoccupation with body image' (Fleming 1989, p.285).

Joy Schaverien

Joy Schaverien, a much-published British art therapist, discusses how food, like art materials, has a physical presence: as a mother provides her child with food, an art therapist offers art materials to her patient. Schaverien notes: 'The concrete nature of this transaction, within the therapeutic boundary, sets up a resonance with the problem.' She concludes: 'Thus it is evident that the relation to the art materials is significant even before a picture is made' (Schaverien 1994, p.36).

Schaverien affirms the traditional transference to the therapist by the anorexic patient as that of the 'controlling parent'. And normally, because of this, the patient would tend to suspend her 'imaginative capacity' to maintain absolute control so as not to be 'overwhelmed'. However, the art therapist's provision of art materials, Schaverien goes on to explain, presents a less traditional alternative: for the patient to begin to 'play' though remaining in control (Wood 1996).

Holly Matto

In her art therapy sessions with eating-disordered patients, Holly Matto challenges them to experiment with a variety of art materials. She explains how changing initial ways of relating to art media can be helpful in tackling dysfunctional belief systems and challenging internal messages like 'I must be perfect in all I do to be worthwhile' or 'I must be in control or I will go crazy'. Matto explains how such messages in the art therapy setting can translate to 'I must create a perfect painting' or 'I can't let myself get too out of control with the paint' (Matto 1997, p.349). She describes how complex it can be to create order out of chaos. It requires 'active decision-making', and involves choosing from endless possibilities: 'Choices might relate to the theme of the piece, the size, the shape, the materials used, the colors used and/or the beginning steps' (p.349).

Matto finds that having patients create collages from images, symbols or words cut out of popular publications is a valuable way to encourage discussion about internalized cultural messages (as generators of dysfunctional thoughts and negative self-statements). Important causes of eating disorders can be confronted directly and in context, making it harder for patients to succumb to traditional self-blaming tendencies.

2. Art-making processes and eating disorders

My approach to art therapy was, in part, generated by two different educational programmes. Dr Martin Fischer at the Toronto Art Therapy Institute was an advocate of spontaneous art-making that offers no directives to patients as to what to make or subject matters on which to focus. However, the instructors at Lesley College, in Cambridge, Massachusetts, taught me the value of giving directives and structure in a session, creating mechanisms for dialogue. Each method has its place in art therapy with eating-disordered patients.

Since control is a major issue in eating disorders, there is much tension around the need to control and for there not to be control. I have found, therefore, among diverse groups of eating-disordered patients, the use of a combination of spontaneous art-making opportunities and specific directives presents individuals with opportunities to act out issues of control and/or lack of it, both on and off the page.

A number of arts therapists have written on the suitability of art-making processes with eating-disordered clients, and the observations of six of them follow here.

Mary Levens

Mary Levens, a British art therapist and pioneering author of publications on art therapy and eating disorders, discusses how art therapy has much to offer eating-disordered patients. Levens notes that for articulate, well-educated patients (which many of them are), intellectualization is a common defence when they are split off from their bodies. Imagery is far less easy to manipulate: creative expression encouraging spontaneity, flexibility and the disclosure of unconscious material (Levens 1987). Wood acknowledges that, during the last decade, Levens has been writing more consistently about her work with people with chronic eating disorders than other therapists:

> She sees the patient's battle with her own body as not only reflecting the experience of it as a bad object, but also as an expression that the patient cannot conceive of her body as a container with an inside and an outside, or as having any boundaries or as taking up any space. For Levens, where the patient does not have a mental 'space', art provides the opportunity to work on these issues through creating a corresponding concrete space. (Wood 1996, p.14)

Also, with respect to therapeutic relationships (and transference), Levens notes that many eating-disordered patients believe that only one person can 'survive a relationship' (Levens 1987, p.3). And, in art-making with all groups of eating-disordered patients, the desire to have one parent to oneself or to put oneself in the middle of them is a recurring theme. Thus, Levens finds that many of her anorexic patients become passive in her presence, projecting their 'power' on to her as therapist.

Mari Fleming

Mari Fleming talks about the art therapist's role in the art therapy process with anorexic patients. Not only does she provide and protect 'safe conditions', but she also serves as a model of ego functioning. By being 'flexible', the art therapist encourages the patient's independent functioning, while still being available to offer guidance: 'As does the "good enough" mother, the art therapist supports the patient's risk taking and solution finding. The art therapist also respects the patient's need to retreat for comfort and soothing by providing structured use of art materials' (Fleming 1989, p.283).

Fleming also notes how, for the anorexic, '[r]efusal to participate in artwork or wishes for merger with the idealized therapist may precipitate defensive withdrawal or attempts to please the therapist' (p.302). Approaches Fleming has developed for bulimics, however, are based on their readiness to both take in and expel. So, Fleming's art group, with anorexic and bulimic members, involved her constant recognition of the anorexic's developmental issues and her need to make adaptations to suit their individual needs.

Ditty Dokter

In the book that she edited, *Arts Therapies and Clients with Eating Disorders: Fragile Board*, Ditty Dokter discusses how psychotherapeutic and art concepts are sometimes seen as mutually exclusive. This is because they use the concept of 'acting out' to dismiss the notion of using the arts as a therapeutic modality. Analysis is seen to practise 'suspended action'; in contrast, the arts therapies practise 'direct action' by means of a particular art modality (Dokter 1994, p.16). Dokter, however, describes patients with eating disorders as an 'acting out client group', acting out their underlying emotional conflicts through the body. She draws attention to the importance of considering how this 'acting out' can be transformed into a 'therapeutic form of action' allowing for internal change.

Though she acknowledges that eating-disordered patients are very well able to think, Dokter doubts their abilities to use verbal reflection and interpretation for personal change, since interpretation in therapy is often experienced as a 'painful re-enactment of being controlled' (p.17). So, she explains ways in which the arts therapies can work on other levels. At the one extreme, anorexics are notorious intellectualizers, making it hard for them to be in touch with their feelings, and, at the other, bulimics feel easily overwhelmed. Art-making processes, therefore, that are neither intellectually demanding nor technically overwhelming can be particularly accommodating to this population's psychotherapeutic needs, offering appropriate 'acting out' opportunities.

Joy Schaverien

Joy Schaverien expands on the 'acting out' theme, in explaining why art psychotherapy is 'potentially effective' in the treatment of patients with eating disorders:

> Art offers an alternative; a way of enacting and symbolizing the inner conflict and it also provides another potential transactional object. Anorexia could be understood to be a form of acting out. *Acting out* behaviour which is motivated by unconscious pain; a form of splitting. The relation to food could be understood to be such acting out. Conversely, *enactment* implies that there is consciousness and so the act has meaning. The art work, as a transactional object, might at first be the channel for unconscious acting out; later, it may develop into an enactment. (Schaverien 1994, p.40)

Explanations of Schaverien's 'transactional object' concept follow in Section 3.

Paola Luzzatto

Paola Luzzatto, a British art therapist, highlights patients talking about their experiences as the final stage of the art therapy process (Wood 1996). Matto states, making reference to Luzzatto: 'Whereas in verbal therapies a client is encouraged to think about past actions, in art therapy a client is encouraged to act first (through symbols/visual metaphors) right in the session and then is encouraged to verbalize such reactions to the experience' (Matto 1997, p.348). And, affirming this, Wood cites Warriner, who stated, towards the end of one year of art therapy, how art therapy helped her 'find her voice through visual language' (Wood 1996, p.17).

Holly Matto

Holly Matto considers an integrated approach for treating eating disorders, presenting an interface between art therapy and cognitive behavioural therapy. She notes how art therapy's provision of space for the creative expression of emotion helps balance out cognitive behavioural therapy approaches:

> Both the art process and the product can help create change in an individual's thought patterns, emotions and behaviors through a variety

of ways. In directly confronting a wide range of emotions such as anger, frustration, joy, gratification, success and failure that inevitably surface during an artistic experience, the subsequent self-statements that go along with such emotions can be addressed, and negative statements can be replaced with more self-enhancing coping statements. In a sense, a client can begin to integrate cognitive understanding and meaning with affective experience. (Matto 1997, pp.348–349)

Matto, referring to Schaverien, also describes the art process and product as helping give dignity to patients' painful emotions, while counteracting the passivity and secrecy attached to their eating disorder:

Anorexic clients tend to begin the therapeutic process in an art therapy session similar to the way they have related to food – extremely selective, controlled and making small marks using a 'safe' medium such as pencil. Bulimic clients, on the other hand, tend to go 'wild' making uncontrollable messes and often ruminating about their creation after they are done, similar to how they have related to food. (p.349)

Matto considers the total effect and significance of the art process for one of her patients:

Art, for Jane, became an empowerment tool by providing her with a means of actively participating in decision-making, enhancing her problem-solving skills and facilitating cognitive insights into her current situation. In addition, her art provided both negative and positive reinforcement by affording Jane the opportunity to express emotions and verbalize her insights and by creating a sense of mastery and control in working hard on her projects. (p.349)

As Michèle Wood points out, most of the British authors who write about the role of the patient's art product, with the possible exception of Schaverien, discuss the importance of paying attention to the dynamics involved in the patient's art-making experience itself (Wood 1996). And she notes how Levens, in her additional role as a psychodramatist, even encourages patients to give non-verbal responses to their images, warning that too early a verbal interpretation can cause concrete thinking to be discarded and 'real experiences' not properly understood.

3. Art products and eating disorders

Art products come in all shapes, sizes and conditions. To some, the art product is everything, and the process of making it of little, if any, value. For others, the making of the product is as significant as the final product itself, maybe even more important. In our product-oriented society, we are very quick to place value on finished products and read purpose or intention into what they may represent or conjure up for us. It is important to ensure, however hard it is where another's art product is concerned, that our viewing should be as projection-free as possible.

Some experts believe that the visual product can simply serve as a concrete way to mark changes and progress. Others, however, offer more complicated explanations about the relevance of art products. Wood (1996) acknowledges that both Schaverien and Murphy see the 'therapeutic agent for change' in art therapy to be the client's communication to herself through unconscious projection into the image when looking at it after making it. Hence, although they both agree on the centrality of the art product, knowing how each gets to the key points may not be as easy.

This is the perfect time to say how much I feel some practitioners' rhetoric can impede the reader's understanding. It is always important to give authority to what we say, especially when there is a variety of opinions on the subject. However, I am convinced the competition to coin new terminology can cause some to lose sight of what they are really talking about. There is nothing like plain English for plain understanding. So, in plain English, the explanation that most writers agree upon is that artwork acts as a buffer between therapist and patient. Briefly stated, in art therapy negative feelings can be directed at the art piece, not at the therapist, both during the art-making process and the subsequent discussion. Therefore, it is easier for the therapist and patient to work together without animosity. I will now go on to relay others' discussions on this.

Mary Levens

Levens draws attention to the way in which the eating-disordered patient and therapist relate to the art object. She states that the anorexic patient who says 'It doesn't mean anything' is sometimes saying 'I'm not going to produce anything for you'. And to ask 'Well, what do you think it is then?' could mean 'I'm not going to work at it – but I'd like to watch you do so' (Levens 1987, p.5).

Levens describes the mishandling of a patient's comments metaphorically. It is like the therapist is 'force-feeding' her with food she cannot possibly digest, because it comes from an external source she is trying to block. Anorexic patients need to discover the meaning of their symbolism for themselves, with minimal therapist input or prompting. Levens advises that anything offered by the therapist should be 'digestible', showing full awareness of what the patient is able to 'take in' herself from her own work, uninfluenced by others.

Mari Fleming

Mari Fleming considers the art product as a 'transitional object' (Fleming 1989). Winnicott was the first to coin this term in 1965. Fleming explains it: in normal development, holding and mirroring functions are gradually transferred from the mother to a transitional object, such as a blanket. This object, which represents the mother, not only provides a sense of security but also can be manipulated by the child. Although cognitively perceived as external, it is still part of the self. Then, as the need-gratifying aspects of the transitional object are gradually internalized, an appropriate self–object response, sense of self and self-esteem start to develop. Fleming cites Winnicott and Edith Kramer, an art therapy pioneer, to explain how art serves as a transitional object:

> Winnicott theorized that the unique value of art in human development and society is in its function as a transitional object, external to the individual but imbued with meaning. Edith Kramer...stated that while art does function as a transitional object, art products are *new* configurations invested with meaning; these art products are not found, but *made*. (Fleming 1989, p.281)

Fleming then provides her own summation:

> To make art, one must initiate action. The artwork made within the treatment process stands for its meaning to the artist and for the relationship with the art therapist. In its function as transitional object, art can provide a corrective experience leading to gradual internalization of soothing and confirming functions. (p.281)

Joy Schaverien

Joy Schaverien gives more complex explanations about the role of the art product for eating-disordered patients. After describing eating-disordered patients' relationship to food as a way of negotiating between their internal world and the environment, she proposes that their completed pictures (or sculptures) negotiate in a similar way to food. This time, however, the negotiation is not only between the inner and outer world of the patient, but between the patient and therapist as well (Schaverien 1994).

In coining and defining the term 'transactional object', Schaverien notes that the art object, as an object of transference itself, may temporarily and unconsciously become a substitute for the use of food. She points out that her view accords with those who consider anorexia to be a borderline disturbance, with pre-symbolic-level functioning. Therefore, if the need for concrete expression can be converted from an obsession with food to a use of art materials, the beginning of a movement towards symbolization can occur.

> Art can offer a means of bringing the anorexic to a stage where she can relate directly to another person. The art process, mediated within the transference, may facilitate a journey from a relatively unconscious, or undifferentiated state, through stages of concrete thinking, to the beginnings of separation and eventually to symbolization. (Schaverien 1994, p.31)

Schaverien comments that treatment can still be successful even if the patient is unable to speak about her pictures. The art medium itself may cause a conscious relationship to unconscious contents to develop, an experience that may later be translated into the spoken word, though this is not essential. As Schaverien says, 'The point is that the patient has the experience of making and owning the pictures and the art therapist is witness to this' (p.31).

Schaverien also explains how, on completion, the picture becomes an object through which unconscious transactions can be made. These involve revealing the significance of the role played by food and the facilitation of interactions with the therapist: through transference, elements of the mother–child feeding relationship may be reproduced.

> The use of food as a transactional object might be understood to be an unconscious displacement of an anxiety or fear. If this displacement can be channelled through art materials it may be possible to bring the original impulse to consciousness. The pictures, as temporary transactional objects, may facilitate the beginning of movement from an unconscious, fused state, where magical thinking is activated, to separation and differentiation. (p.37)

Schaverien goes on to describe how access to the picture is controlled by the artist, the picture becoming, like food, 'a private matter'. It is also an object through which to negotiate 'mediation for control' without the necessity of verbal intervention.

> A picture creates space and it offers a way of potentially sharing that space by permitting the imaginal world to be viewed. The anorexic does not usually permit herself imaginal space; she does not dare to dream or risk chaos; nor can she permit her vigilance to lapse for a moment. She fears mess and intrusion and by either she may be overwhelmed. A picture, even the first tentative attempts of the anorexic, permits the possibility of contained mess, within the framed space of the picture. Here chaos may be held safely within the boundaries of the paper, separated from its creator, and it may exhibit the imaginal world. (p.41)

Schaverien also describes the picture as a 'scapegoat', in that it can embody chaos and feared aspects of the inner world:

> On the paper these may become 'live' within the therapeutic relationship. Here the client may engage in a way in which she cannot dare to venture to engage with the therapist ... Simultaneously, the picture protects the transitional area; it keeps the space between patient and therapist. (p.41)

Schaverien brings her various explanations together in a surprisingly simple summative paragraph:

> The pictures facilitate a relationship, first to the self, and then to another person; in this way they begin to embody some of the power which was previously invested in food and so they become transactional objects in place of food. The therapist is present as witness; and so it is likely that the relation to the therapist may repeat some of the power which was invested in the parents. (p.46)

Unfortunately, Schaverien's narrative, though important, is complicated: it is too detailed and unclear for many. Wood is quite sceptical about the 'transactional object'. She does not feel that it adequately describes what the therapist actually exchanges in the transaction with the client, and states: 'In my opinion the transactional object is a very limited explanation for the role and function of the client's art work in therapy' (Wood 1996, p.18).

Paola Luzzatto

Art therapist Paola Luzzatto has written about the 'double trap' of anorexic patients. She has observed the prevalence of three types of imagery in their artwork: a 'victim' (either imprisoned or cornered), a 'trap' (either imprisoning or cornering the victim) and a 'bad object' (ready to attack or reject the victim, should she attempt escape from the trap) (Luzzatto 1994). Luzzatto states that though different patients may depict this imagery in different ways, there are significant commonalities. First, the 'victim' usually appears as immature, fragile and almost boneless and sexless. Second, the 'trap' appears to be containing the victim, and is usually in the form of a fish bowl, circle of persecutors or corner of a room. Finally, the persecution from a 'bad object' is usually represented by various threats: being imprisoned and inhibited, engulfed and annihilated, or rejected and punished.

Discussing the psychodynamic nature of her approach, Luzzatto states: 'The image of the double trap may be seen to represent a basic internalized object-relationship of these patients and their emotional position toward themselves and toward the world' (p.141). So, Luzzatto sees it as her responsibility, as art therapist, to help the patient recognize that her internal pattern (as projected in her imagery) is projected on to the outside world all the time. This makes others, including the therapist, appear aggressive and rejective of them.

Luzzatto also describes a kind of 'paradoxical communication': 'I need you – but you must not help me.' Seeing that a subgroup of anorexic patients have internal worlds that do not contain an internalized good object, she realizes how frightening their external worlds must be and why they make 'defensive immobility' a chief survival mechanism. According to Wood (1996), Luzzatto acknowledges more directly than other writers on the subject the anorexic client's desperate unwillingness to change. She explains how art therapy helps facilitate change in the patient's perception of her internal world, as well as allowing for interactive capacities with the external world to be enhanced.

Like that of Levens, Luzzatto's theoretical basis for understanding the client is a psychoanalytic object relations one, and her construction of 'the double trap' (a formulation of theory from practice) helps introduce her concept of 'double transference'. Art therapy's significance for Luzzatto lies in the possibilities it permits for 'double transference', enabling more positive interactions to ensue between patient and therapist. Wood (1996) believes that Luzzatto's explanations of the 'double trap' and 'double transference' provide a clear framework with which to think about and construct clinical practice. Though critical of Schaverien's 'transactional object', Wood makes positive comparisons between Luzzatto's 'double transference' and

Schaverien's 'scapegoat transference'. Both allow for positive projection on to the therapist and negative projection on to the image.

4. Art therapy with anorexic patients

The anorexic patient is not only emotionally restricted because of her condition, but also physically starved, which compounds responses to treatment. The ability to concentrate and process gets her off to a tentative start with art-making. Four art therapists have written significantly on the subject – Diane Mitchell, Diane Waller, June Murphy and Mary Levens.

Diane Mitchell

According to the American art therapist Diane Mitchell, Bruch (one of the most respected early researchers on eating disorders), among others, has used art therapy in the treatment of anorexia with significant results. For Mitchell, the fact that the anorexic inaccurately perceives or conceptualizes can often be associated with her inability to communicate with others. Communication difficulties with others may play out in several ways: from an abiding sense of loneliness, to a feeling of not being respected by others, to a hypersensitivity to insult and abuse (Mitchell 1980).

Mitchell explains how art therapy provides the withdrawn anorexic, who is unable to experience what she is feeling, with the opportunity to share with others what is going on for her through her painting. With the help of a skilled art therapist, the creative act itself, consideration of expressed theme(s) and understanding through therapeutic processing can all draw attention to emerging unconscious conflicts that can then be dealt with appropriately.

Mitchell also discusses how, in art therapy, the 'control' that the anorexic values so much can actually be worked with, not against: 'The patient has complete control of the media to use however she wants and the chance to verbalize as she chooses about her painting. What she creates is her own graphic projection, and she alone can answer for it' (p.58). The skilled art therapist, also, can go beyond what the patient has said by interpreting, in a non-threatening manner, what she feels might be trying to be expressed. Mitchell recommends that initial art therapy sessions with the anorexic patient should be directive-free, so that she feels comfortable enough to freely express herself in this modality. She also recommends that detailed questioning of the patient about herself or her artwork should be avoided.

Mitchell goes on to list individual directives that can be given once a relationship develops between the patient and therapist. She suggests that the directives selected relate to the patient's therapeutic goals and objectives. Here are some of them:

1. draw yourself (self-projection of body image)

2. draw yourself as you would like to be (conceptualization of self in future)

3. draw your family or members of your family separately (discussing feelings about family, relationships, interactions and conflicts)

4. draw how you are feeling abstractly (using colours, shapes and designs to represent emotions)

5. draw the path or course of your life

6. graphically portray emotions (such as anger, sorrow, loneliness, love, peace and happiness)

7. draw what you would like the future to hold for you.

Diane Waller and the Goldsmiths' College study

The Goldsmiths' College study (Waller 1981) was initiated by Diane Waller 'to investigate the effectiveness of art/psychotherapy as a treatment for sufferers of eating disorders such as anorexia nervosa and obesity' (Murphy 1984, p.103). Since most of the subjects were experiencing body image distortion, certain techniques to facilitate an awareness of actual body size and a more realistic self-image were key in the investigation. A series of exercises that concentrated on certain parts of the body were included. These involved using video, masks and make-up, as well as paintings of an ideal self and a group activity to make life-size models that acted as their 'other' selves.

The study noted that anorexics rarely drew the human figure in any of their artwork and seemed to experience difficulty if asked to do so. It was suggested that this may be connected with their distorted body image. When figures did appear, they were usually either long, thin and boy-like or caricatured; for example, a doll-like girl with long hair and a narrow waist, standing in a bed of flowers. This could be seen as a portrayal of an 'idealized self' rooted in the anorexic's failure to accept her real sexual identity (Murphy 1984, p.103).

The Goldsmiths' College study also revealed that many of the paintings reflected the anorexic's 'stark social environment', both within the family and her social interactions beyond it. More often than not, the paintings portrayed images of isolation, and frequently indicated that the patient had been bullied or ridiculed at some stage in her life. The general isolation from fellow members of the anorexic's peer group became more obvious in the art group situation: a real fear of participation was combined with a genuine inability to express inner feelings.

One of the most significant findings to emerge from the study concerns the consistency of recurrent imagery spontaneously produced in the individual sessions. Murphy recorded that they seemed to fall into four category headings or thematic groups:

1. concise extrinsic patterns; for example, whirlpools and bottomless pits
2. animals, usually dogs and horses
3. flowers and plants, cacti and thorns
4. landscapes and gardens. (p.104)

The study noted how these four categories corresponded to the different stages of therapy, showing a progression towards more expressive imagery. Then, usually after more open imagery developed, there was a return to drawing concise patterns, indicating feelings of despair about being trapped in an insoluble situation. Consequently, some regressive behaviour followed: there was a return to being defensive and 'acting out', including refusing to eat and obsessional behaviour like 'ritual washing'.

The study also offered interpretations for each of the individual categories. Category one, the intricate patterns and vortices, could indicate the anorexic's barriers in personal expression and human involvement. Category two, the dogs and horses, could reflect the anorexic's urge for exercise, which ties in with her overactivity and lack of fatigue. Category three, the variety of plant forms (drawn spontaneously and with general competence and great attention to detail), could indicate how the anorexic perceives herself. The landscapes and trees of category four were viewed in Jungian terms as 'archetypal configurations'.

June Murphy

June Murphy, a British art therapist who wrote about the Goldsmiths' College study, also wrote about her own use of art therapy in the treatment of anorexia nervosa. In Britain in the early 1980s, approximately one in every two hundred adolescent girls was alleged to be anorexic to some degree.

Murphy's writing stems from her notes and observations about her own experiences working with adolescent patients over a four-year period. Under the heading 'Art therapy: A new dimension in the treatment of anorexia nervosa', Murphy highlights the aspects of art therapy that make it more appropriate as a treatment process than traditional methods. Placing the emphasis on a painting removes the focus from the patient in an intensive psychotherapeutic relationship, providing a less threatening and safer environment for intensive therapy to take place (Murphy 1984).

Since pictures facilitate personal exploration (e.g. fantasies and self-image) while providing a safe vent for feelings (e.g. anger, depression and fear), they can shed light on relationships as well as other 'ambivalent' feelings (central in most adolescent experience). Murphy lists specific issues confronted by the adolescent anorexic: 'Her difficulties in personal relationships, particularly with her mother; preoccupations with self-image, thinness, bodily functions; and obsessions and fads in eating and other maladjustment in behaviour' (Murphy 1984, p.100).

She goes on to emphasize that one of the most important aspects of art therapy is that the patient must actively participate in her own treatment – and recovery. In verbal therapy, long periods of silence are traditional, and often exacerbate a sense of despair and helplessness: 'The actual painting process helps break down defensive/defiant responses that often block early stages of treatment' (p.101).

Murphy states: 'The initial commitment to paper is a statement of commitment to therapy' (p.101). And, through expression on paper, the confusion and ambivalence that the anorexic usually tries to conceal about her sense of identity are externalized and clarified. Murphy discusses how identity crises are experienced by many adolescents. However, for anorexics, she notes, they are made worse since they are masked by the more visible physical and psychological symptoms of their more apparent primary disorder.

Murphy explains that since anorexics have usually been told how they feel, a more traditional interpretive approach is not helpful in solving their identity crisis. Through art therapy, however, the 'tangible products' expressed by the anorexic help to reveal that she has feelings of her own, even though they might be hidden and confused. (A painting is unique to the individual who has made it, and 'belongs' to her.) Murphy refers to Jung to elaborate and confirm how the patient can make herself creatively independent through painting. No longer dependent on her dreams or doctor's knowledge, she gives herself shape by painting herself. Then, in discussing the painting or art form with the art therapist, the patient can become aware of her confusion, and hopefully work towards a clearer sense of self.

As a cathartic experience, the painting process allows emotions to be released and defensive barriers to be broken down. For the anorexic, the issue of control is central: she wants to remain in control of herself and attempts to control other people by preventing them controlling her. The fear of losing control can, in some cases, be equivalent to the fear of losing her whole existence. So, starting to paint can represent a bold step into the unknown: the anorexic's fear of it is the main reason for resistance to participation in art therapy. However, Murphy is quick to point out how the patient can also use the painting experience to learn mastery and control, first of images on paper. Later, this can lead to a sense of security and an exploration of the issue of needing to be in control. She states: 'Only by losing control can the learning experience of regaining it be achieved' (p.102).

Murphy also explains that the anorexic's anxiety about losing control is so strong that it causes her to build inflexible defence mechanisms. Because painting is an unfamiliar means of expression, it has the power to shift formerly fixed barriers and makes the patient aware of her defences. However, there is always the chance that the patient will learn how to prevent 'exposing' herself through her artwork by adapting her defences. Although this seldom happens, Murphy points out that the art therapist must be skilled enough to understand the anorexic's need to 'adjust' and work with it constructively. Owing to the anorexic's general defensiveness, Murphy suggests the early stages of art therapy treatment be non-directive. Once the patient has been allowed to work at her own pace, within the boundaries of a 'safe' environment and a 'flexible' relationship, initial trust is established. Then, the difficult task of identifying and getting in touch with feelings can begin.

Mary Levens

Wood explains how Mary Levens's work with anorexic patients goes one stage beyond Murphy's. Instead of viewing artwork as mirroring the anorexic's experiences through content, she emphasizes the connection between the use of art materials and the experience of bodily sensations (Wood 1996). Levens also refrains from her usually non-directive approach to art therapy with patients in the early stages of treatment, who she feels often need more direction. Again, unlike Murphy, Levens suggests themes for them to focus on, commenting: 'This lack of self-direction and autonomy may be regarded as an important part of their psychopathology' (Levens 1987, p.3).

Levens illustrates how starved patients can often deal more directly with actual concrete experiences through art-making, and chooses the example of 18-year-old Katy to show how art-making can frequently be linked, symbolically, to bodily experiences. Katy painted an image of herself in white on white paper, effectively making herself invisible. Commenting on Katy's process, Levens explains how beginning to express something 'real' for herself was terrifying. This was a young woman who felt that her mother had always exactly known how she felt and what she thought, making her 'transparent' within her family. Katy obviously felt that by remaining invisible on the paper others would be less able to control her (Levens 1987).

Levens also discusses how art therapy works for anorexic patients because it is not about 'getting something right' (a common obsession). And relating to an object instead of a person can conjure up feelings of flexibility not usually present in direct communication.

5. Art therapy with bulimic patients

The bulimic patient is all over the place, physically and emotionally, and so is her art-making. Her responses to treatment are complicated by her fluctuations in mood, motivation and damaged and confused senses of appropriateness. A number of art therapists and others have made important contributions to the literature on the subject. I have included overviews of the work of several of them here.

Andrea Morenoff and Barbara Sobol

American clinicians Andrea Morenoff (social worker) and Barbara Sobol (art therapist) describe their art therapy approach to the long-term psychodynamic treatment of bulimic women. They believe that their work is most effective when it takes place in a group setting. This is because the setting affects their pacing, preventing a process that may become too threatening because it moves too quickly. And, as in all group work, patients' processes are enhanced and supported through observations of each other's ways and with feedbacks (Morenoff and Sobol 1989). Morenoff and Sobol point out where group art therapy differs from other therapy groups. Referring to Ulman, they describe how the act of creation is essentially 'a solitary act', with the first audience being an audience of one – the artist herself. Making art in a group, however, allows individuals to include others in 'private creative experiences'.

Morenoff and Sobol keep art assignments general enough to be applicable at almost any phase of therapy. They feel that by giving simple instructions that are open to interpretation there is little offered to the patient around which cognitive response can be structured:

> To elicit authentic self-expression, therapists should create a setting and an expectation that invite the client to engage and invest freely in the artwork. This means providing ample space and time, minimizing distractions, and offering appropriate reassurance that any effort will be respected and accepted (Morenoff and Sobol 1989, p.164).

Morenoff and Sobol also suggest assignments should provide support for the individual's developmental needs. For instance, themes concerning what is most currently painful to patients, such as their isolation or sense of shame in their relationship to food, require greater ego strength. And art products should not be critiqued, with the therapists modelling appropriate responses for the group:

> Oftentimes, images that may be disturbing are not described or acknowledged (or even recognized) by the client. In our treatment model the therapist is advised to respect that avoidance. When unduly disturbing or provocative images are presented, it is the responsibility of the therapist to respond with caution and to pay attention to the client's expressed or implied need to keep what is still unmanageable (even though graphically expressed) at a preconscious level. This can be done by actively focusing on a positive aspect of the image, thereby creating a more balanced internal perception. (p.165)

Morenoff and Sobol also discuss how art tasks can elicit primary process material. So, they extend the invitation for patients 'overly stimulated' by their own disturbing imagery – to produce artworks that are soothing and supportive of the self.

Mary Levens

Mary Levens discusses how bulimic patients often describe the fantasy of eating paint:

> The very act of painting appears to encourage associations to do with taking things in and vomiting things out. They frequently create 'smear'

or 'mess' paintings, with finger paints or dollops of thick poster paint, and describe their using these materials, as if the contents of their bodies, blood, vomit, faeces, were spilling out onto the paper. (Levens 1987, p.3)

Levens goes on to give the example of 25-year-old Sandra, a bulimic patient who has painted a 'vomit picture' that she described as more real than herself. Levens comments on the tremendous sense of relief Sandra feels and the vast amount of paper, paint and space used. According to Levens, the use of art-making as an alternative way to empty herself of feelings is not what should become important to Sandra. For the activity to promote some internal change (and defensive actions not to be repeated), both patient and therapist need to be actively involved in understanding what happens, as it happens.

This example causes Levens to talk about 'enactment' as opposed to 'acting out' behaviours (Schaverien: see Section 2), and how only the former can be therapeutic. Wood draws attention to Levens's caution that if the art therapist does not recognize the difference between 'enactment' and 'acting out' behaviour, as manifested non-verbally in the artwork, eating-disordered behaviours may be, inadvertently, reinforced and stimulated. Wood states: 'For Levens art therapy can facilitate self-awareness in a total way, particularly by providing an experience for the patient of inhabiting their bodies' (Wood 1996, p.14).

Levens also notes how bingeing anorexic and bulimic patients are usually more in touch with their bodies and issues to do with their sexuality. This is why they often create images of menstruation, self-disgust at their female parts and the lack of control that they have over them (Levens 1987).

Jacqueline Gillespie

Jacqueline Gillespie is an American psychologist who discusses how bulimics are often referred to as 'failed anorexics' (Gillespie 1996). However, she notes that they have their own set of issues. While they are extremely careful about monitoring and maintaining their weight in response to social pressures, exhibiting similar control behaviours to anorexics, they usually lack obsessions with thinness and disturbed self-perceptions. So, their drawings of people tend to be hyper-realistic, emphasizing females with perfect bodies and elaborate clothing.

6. Art therapy and body image

Body image concerns affect most of us, whether or not we have an eating disorder. Diane Mitchell focuses on anorexia nervosa as representing 'a pathetic illustration of the confused attitudes induced by society idolizing certain body images for all of us' (Mitchell 1980, p.57). Condemned to the 'torture of self-starvation', the anorexic displays 'the futile hope of "deserving" respect and gaining praise and recognition for being so thin' (p.57).

Some of us dress cleverly to cover up our shape and size, while others flaunt what we have: body image concerns can both precipitate and perpetuate eating disorders. Arts therapists and non-arts therapists have written extensively on the subject.

Irma Dosamantes

Irma Dosamantes, an American dance/movement therapist, in her article 'Body-image: Repository for cultural idealizations and denigrations of the self', discusses how each culture appears to have some idealized body image that is shared by most of its members. Preferred body images alter in reaction to our environment: we mould our bodies unconsciously, according to our experiences. The present dominant culture in the United States favours the youthful, slender, physically fit body and western European facial features. In Dosamantes's words, 'We are a culture in search of an unattainable perfection' (Dosamantes 1992, p.266).

Dosamantes also points out that although there is no necessary correlation between the way we and others perceive our bodies, how satisfied we are with our physical appearance is dependent on how well we like ourselves. She states: 'Negative attitudes toward the body frequently manifest themselves in the avoidance and denial of particular body parts or types of body images.' She cites anorexics' need to be 'exceedingly thin' as an important part of their body image. And, when they are not, she remarks that, according to Cooper and Fairburn, '[t]hey are likely to consider themselves weak, lazy, unlovable and incompetent' (p.258). Art therapy obviously plays an important role in helping eating-disordered patients identify their distorted body image perceptions and related considerations, as well as facilitating possibilities for change.

Nadine Kaslow and Virginia Eicher

American authors Nadine Kaslow (psychologist) and Virginia Eicher (dance and drama therapist), in their article 'Body image therapy: A combined creative arts therapy and verbal psychotherapy approach', describe a clay-making technique used by Wooley and Wooley. This involves the creation of a series of clay sculptures in which patients make representations of their bodies in several conditions: as they are now, as they were before being anorexic and as they might be imagined in the future (Kaslow and Eicher 1988). This exercise can also be done using drawing and painting materials. Its purpose is to increase expression of feelings about the body and body image distortions, as well as to lead to improved reality testing, which acknowledges the flexibility of body image perceptions.

As well as being concerned with individual patients' considerations of their own body images, Kaslow and Eicher recognize the importance of 'family body image' exercises. They explain how it is hard for the eating-disordered patient not to be affected or influenced by the bodies of significant others around her. Several directives are suggested that might be useful for exploring related issues: Wooley and Wooley's abstract collage using geometric shapes to represent family members; Kinetic Family Draw-ings (especially with family members involved in eating situations); and choosing objects in the room to represent family members, placing them in relation to one another.

It is Kaslow and Eicher's belief that by directly focusing on body image issues, more rapid and complete recovery from eating disorders is possible. They support patients in their growing awareness of the body as a separate or transitional object (referring to Sugarman and Kurash 1982), noting that it is essential for the body to develop into a positive object in order for a healthy process of separation/individuation to occur.

Jacqueline Gillespie

Jacqueline Gillespie talks about the quandary of working with eating-disordered patients in verbal modalities. This is because the disordered perceptions of the body that are often their main focus are described in concrete pictorial terms. Accordingly, she feels that art therapists are 'uniq-uely positioned' to go beyond the talk surrounding concerns about the body and associated self issues, making visual representations in paint or clay (Gillespie 1996).

7. Art therapy with abused patients

The abused patient transfers much repressed trauma directly on to the page or into the clay. She is comforted and enraged, in painful and prolific bouts, by means that verbal therapy sessions cannot provide. An increasing number of art therapists have made important contributions to the literature on the subject. Here I focus on three.

Sandra Ticen

According to Sandra Ticen, an American art therapist, over 50 per cent of eating-disordered patients have experienced some form of sexual trauma. Her article 'Feed me … Cleanse me … Sexual trauma projected in the art of bulimics' discusses how the bulimic patient needs 'a safe, structured place to grieve and recreate her purging metaphor' (Ticen 1987, p.17). Art therapy is seen to be able to provide this.

Ticen explains how eating disorders may be triggered by traumatic events. Since a preoccupation with food is less disturbing than the intrusive thoughts of trauma, victims give themselves a sense of control through it. She notes that the more traumatized the victim, the more restricted the art will be, and affirms: 'With consistent, ongoing abreactive work in art therapy, the imagery will gradually become more fluid, more colorful, more integrated and more dynamic' (p.18). Art therapy's adaptive method enables the patient to symbolically 'binge–purge' and 'mess–cleanse'.

Ticen has found that there are few differences in working with the sexually abused anorexic and sexually abused bulimic. Nevertheless, she notes that, depending on the severity of the traumatization, the bulimic patient will often take more risks, reaching treatment goals more quickly. Since most bulimics are not as nutritionally deficient as anorexics, their cognitive processes are usually clearer, permitting faster recovery patterns, both physiologically and psychologically.

Ticen refers to Golub when stating how art therapy provides the abused patient with a method of sublimation while offering an extension between self and trauma. However, she warns: 'Working abreactively with the victim of sexual abuse, the therapist must attempt to regulate the flow of affect if it appears that the imagery may flood the ego, causing the patient to feel more out of control' (p.20). Ticen emphasizes the bulimic's very weak ego boundaries. This makes the therapist's task very delicate, having to know what media to offer and when to intervene, without taking control or being intrusive, which can make for a very slow process. She describes 'one of the most paralyzing effects of sexual abuse' as being seen in the art projections of the self. And, for the bulimic, the distortion may not be so much related to size as to worth.

Carolyn S. Waller

Carolyn S. Waller, an American art therapist, discusses how art therapy with a group of adult female incest survivors increases the value of catharsis, cohesion and insight as curative factors in their treatment (Waller 1992). In Waller's art therapy group, catharsis was performed in two ways: through the use of the art medium and through the verbalizations of strong and long-repressed emotions.

Cohesion came about though the sharing of art materials as well as the sharing of common problems and experiences, and the knowledge that another had had a similar history encouraged closeness among group members. Insight into the origins and present effects of serious problems could be accelerated by sharing the insights of another woman with a similar problem. Thus, examining a problem became a concrete event through the visual expression of that problem and its possible solutions, and feedback from trusted others. For the clients, the art product acted as some sort of buffer between themselves and the world, since they could raise or lower barriers through it, at will, depending on how threatening the contents were to them.

Cathy Malchiodi

Cathy Malchiodi, a pioneer in American art therapy, discusses how many therapists imagine that traumatized children will create art expressions that depict violent and abusive scenes in vivid detail, but this is not usually the case. Not only is the traumatizing event not always drawn, but details in structural elements such as line quality and content are sparse, and colours often limited to black and/or red. And since images are frequently drawn quickly, little attention is given to detail, with poorly integrated or composed figures often resembling stereotyped cartoons or doodles (Malchiodi 1998). I find much correlation here between the art depictions of traumatized children and those eating-disordered patients who have been abused.

When eating-disordered patients start in the art therapy group, those who have made art before are often intimidated because they feel they have to impress, and those who are uncomfortable with making art can be extremely frustrated and resistant. However, it is evident that fears and aversions seem to dissipate after a short while because art is not being made for product, and self-discoveries are facilitated with ease and by surprise in a safe and nurturing environment.

CHAPTER 4

Poetry Therapy and Eating Disorders

1. Principles

The focus of my PhD research was on the integration of poetry in psycho-therapeutic practice. Here, I devoted a lot of time to looking back over my own spontaneously written poetry, which I described as 'wordscapes', and to considering its healing properties (Makin 1998). I had written a variety of pieces over a thirteen-year period, mostly at times of difficulty, which seemed to soothe me and clarify situations. Just as with art therapy, at the time when I started doing it for my own self-care, I thought that I was on to something: that I had invented a therapeutic technique which could be helpful to other people as well, at their difficult times.

It was not long before I learned that what I was doing spontaneously had already been converted into a professional practice, that the National Association for Poetry Therapy (NAPT) existed in the United States, and that there were guidelines, standards and even training offered in this field. Many clinicians, however, are still unaware of, or feel less need for, such an organization, and apply their own brands of poetry therapy in their work. Once I had discovered NAPT, I saw it to be a supportive body, and decided to 'play by the rules' and fees! So, after embarking on the approved training programme to learn correct and expanded ways of working with poetry in psychotherapeutic treatment, I slowly started to integrate what I was learning into my work with eating-disordered patients.

Very little has been written about the use of poetry therapy with eating disorders, apart from a book chapter by psychologists Camay Woodall and Arnold Anderson. Here, they discuss their work using poetry therapy with anorexic patients (Woodall and Anderson 1989). A refusal to speak – and eat – in anorexics is traced back to difficulties in mother–infant vocalization during nursing, where the infant has been unable to indicate her feelings or have them understood.

Woodall and Anderson also consider 'unevenness of development'. Despite frequently having high IQs and levels of academic achievement, anorexics are not often creative or divergent thinkers. Although unable to look at a problem from a variety of angles, they can still memorize and reproduce complex course work. Thus, when it comes to emotions, their alexithymic tendencies are demonstrated by limited vocabulary usage, even numbness, showing repressed affect. Demonstrations of detached, controlled, intellectual stances and cognitive achievements mask abandoned feelings.

Taking into account the anorexic's perceptual and cognitive obstacles, Woodall and Anderson prescribe the introduction of the use of metaphor as remedy: 'Since body experience and the experience of feelings are pre-verbal in origin and often not conscious, they may best be approached through the use of metaphor, which depends on body experience but is expressed verbally' (Woodall and Anderson 1989, p.193).

Poetry therapy for purposes of emotional growth, as described by Woodall and Anderson, can be carried out in two main stages: first, with a poem relevant to the patient's condition being selected, read and interpreted by the therapist; second, with the patient writing a poem based on a significant theme also thought suitable by the therapist. Woodall and Anderson's account of key poetry therapy techniques, as well as not being all-encompassing (as they themselves acknowledge), also suggests a little more control and projection by the therapist than I am comfortable working with. It is important to note that there are many other ways of carrying out poetry therapy, offering more flexibility for the patient (Makin 1998). However, I wish to discuss Woodall and Anderson's explanations of their work in context here, and review it accordingly.

Their rationale for using poetry therapy in the treatment of anorexics focuses on its capacity to aid in assertiveness and expressiveness. In the poetry therapy processes that they use with anorexics, they note: 'Reticence gives way to the interest in a cognitive task (which ends up full of feeling), and the spontaneous poem itself becomes an emergent self-assertion' (Woodall and Anderson 1989, p.194). They also comment that the patient who finds it difficult to speak directly to the therapist will often accept a writing task, which, ironically, has the same end – enabling the patient to relate pertinent information to the therapist. They continue: '… the therapist is then provided with substantial material to discuss and interpret, and the patient is gently confronted with original metaphors she can accept as coming from her own, perhaps previously buried, feelings' (p.194).

Woodall and Anderson recommend the poetry of Emily Dickinson (1830–1885) as particularly relevant to the anorexic population. Emily Dickinson was a college-educated woman who returned to her parents' home and never married. For the most part, she lived a secluded existence, was a perfectionist and had much self-control. Therefore, her poetry includes many feelings connected with loneliness, isolation, depression, frightening images, separation issues, anger, disillusionment and even food restriction.

Woodall and Anderson describe their methodology in sessions incorporating Dickinson's work:

> The therapist presents a poem about loneliness before one about anger, assuming that anger is a more threatening emotion for the anorexic than loneliness. A poem about psychological integration is not presented before the person has a chance to express grief. Also, a patient and therapist can spend more than one session with one of the poems. Indeed, this is indicated when the patient's original poem in response to one of Dickinson's is rich in detail or is so meaningful that both she and the therapist do not wish to go on to the next poem in the sequence. The meaning in the poem is often provided by the original metaphors that the patients produce. The metaphors structurally contain a known (to the reader) physical half and an unknown psychological half... (p.195)

Woodall and Anderson also discuss key poetry therapy principles for poem selection: 'Works that are too sophisticated or long tend to discourage the reticent patient from the task of discovering and putting her own feelings into words. For poetry therapy, a poem should be concise, about deeply personal issues, and of an empowering tone' (p.195).

The anorexic patient's original poem is looked at by Woodall and Anderson for its provision of rich experiential data. Often containing images from her early life and of her family, the poem can reveal feelings of excitement, grief, longing, fear and guilt. Born in a moment of deep introspection, primed by the experience of another writer with whom the patient can identify, this poem is the patient's own production, not a theory, technique or bias. Thus, her fear of being controlled from without is lessened with this approach; the poem becomes the vehicle for enhanced self-esteem.

Woodall and Anderson also note how the use of poetry therapy with anorexic patients can prevent intellectualized discussions that often jeopardize conventional verbal sessions: avoidance of the identification of basic emotional states through censoring and self-interrupting styles is not possible. They then go on to their three main reasons for using poetry therapy:

1. as a short-term intervention, significant change has been found in as few as ten sessions

2. as an adjunct to conventional insight-oriented approaches, a means of breaking through initial resistances is offered, emphasizing the formulation and focusing of thoughts through connecting with creative discoveries

3. there are no obvious dangers.

The last point is emphasized with a quote from Jack Leedy, a poetry therapy pioneer: 'No one has ever died from too much poetry.' Woodall and Anderson do remind the reader, however, that successful poetry therapy does ultimately rely on the therapist's skill and training.

In looking more closely at how poetry therapy actually works with anorexic patients, Woodall and Anderson come up with six ways. They follow here with my comments in parentheses:

1. A poem is seen as an invariable communication which allows contact with another person in a non-threatening way, particularly if it is published. The anorexic, in particular, is very relieved not to have to talk directly to the therapist.

2. A writing task can cause a patient to turn off her conscious defences and connect with feelings in a non-obvious way. This helps lower the barriers between therapist and patient, lessening authority and control issues. (These are key blocks in therapy with anorexics.)

3. A well-chosen poem can not only cause a patient to identify with the conflicts stated in it, but also to experience relief vicariously. Then, in turn, the patient may be encouraged to make formulations about what her own issues could concern. (Anorexics need as many opportunities as possible to make their *own* formulations.)

4. Comparisons are made between the poetic process and symptom formation; initial ideas and inspirations in poetry-making being compared to impulses or conflicts contributing to symptom formation. The act of making a poem, however, causes

communication, even if the meaning of a symptom is unknown. (For anorexics, poetry provides a means of transforming into words what is communicated through physical symptoms.)

5. Being proud of academic accomplishment can be transferred to being proud of a poem, which helps increase self-esteem. So, what would usually be painful realizations are mollified by the pride of accomplishment. (This is something that the anorexic needs to be able to feel authentically.)

6. The patient's poem is *not* an interpretation of behavior or part of a theory. It is her own creation that actually acts as a bridge. This is from the reticent self, to the therapist, to her own healthy self. (The anorexic may thus realize that the therapist is working *with* her, not imposing on her.)

In closing, Woodall and Anderson turn to Winnicott, who stated: 'A poem is layer upon layer of meaning ... and always about the self.'

2. Practices

In the article 'A tale of eating: Writing as a pathway out of an eating disorder', Fiona Place tells her own story. She discusses how one of the most important needs of a person with an eating disorder is to find her own voice, and to be able to describe experiences in her own words, rather than 'the restrictive narrative of an eating problem' (Place 1994, p.189). For her, creative writing was not only helpful in opening up her closed narrative but also in enabling her to see the value of eliciting reflective, as well as affective, responses.

In my group work with eating-disordered patients, I provide many opportunities, usually at the start of sessions as warm-up exercises, for patients to use their own words. And even when subject matters included in directives are broad, not related to an eating disorder, they more often than not still find their way back to one. Whatever is most prominent on a person's mind will invariably fuel their written, as well as spoken, words and artwork.

Often, patients have handed me poems that they have written spontaneously between groups. I will now share these with you, from two patients. The first three poems were written by Deborah, an anorexic in her mid-40s, whose eating disorder started after she sustained a closed head injury in a motor vehicle accident. Since her house had burned down a few years prior to the accident, it was even harder for her to rebuild her memories, not having photographs and familiar possessions around her. Thus, she felt deeply out of control. She went from being highly active and sociable to not wishing to go out. Nevertheless, her strong sense of humour remained undiminished, and though that is not reflected in the poems that follow, it was a very powerful asset, both for herself and other group members.

Although art and writing were not Deborah's modalities of choice prior to being injured, they soon became important components in her self-help and recovery. When Deborah did speak up in verbal groups, her timing and content were not always appropriate, irritating other group members. And because of how her responses were received, it soon became hard for her to say anything at all. However, her written poetry, which was honest, clear, spontaneous, well-timed and appropriate, was easier for her to produce and more enthusiastically received. She could be who she was on the page; however sad what she had to say was for herself and others to hear. Although the focus of Deborah's treatment was on her eating disorder, it became obvious from her poetry that more time really needed to be spent on issues more directly related to her head injury. Deborah's poems follow here.

Feelings

I keep my feelings bottled up for a while
Whenever I'm sad, I laugh and I smile
I don't feel the love that I want to feel
I always feel lonely and my life seems too real.

I don't act how I feel and it feels like a lie
I tell jokes and I laugh when I really want to cry.

This doesn't work and it doesn't feel good
Act how I feel? I would if I could!
So I'll just sit here with no place to go
Asking questions with answers that I'll never know.

Mirror

I was looking at a statue and compared it to myself,
It looked lonely and sad as it sat there on the shelf.
And I could have sworn I saw a tear,
Rolling on its hard cold beard,
And I could have sworn I heard it say,
'Excuse me sir, would you like to stay?'

It's no fun being made of stone,
Sitting on a shelf all alone.
Everyone thinks I feel no pain,
I'm just a statue without a name.
And then I thought how I feel great,
Finally someone to whom I could relate.

I watch people walk by me and they don't see,
There's a lovely person inside of me,
Some days go slow and others fast,
But this face of stone is just a mask.
Believe it or not, my feelings are real,
But my facial expression doesn't show how I feel.

And then I rubbed my eyes to see,
That lonely statue was really me.

Nothing

My life is left without a destination
Lifeless dreams and empty inspiration
In a soul-searching investigation
I find nothing.

My heart is empty, my dreams are dead
There's been no meaning in the words I've said
And as I sift through my cluttered head
I find nothing.

Nothing out there to which I can relate
Nothing left to anticipate
I search and search to find something great
I find nothing.

I look and look as far as I can see
Look deep into eternity.
Became lost in mediocracy
With nothing.

The next four poems were written by Margaret, a 22-year-old patient with an eight-year history of restricting anorexia. Her focus in the first three is entirely on her eating disorder and how it makes, or has made, her feel. Poem four, written to the programme team, heralds her discharge from the hospital and recovery.

Red Light, Green Light

I see her walking up the street each day
And find myself staring as I slow too by the red.

There are others like her
But not many.
She stands out in the crowd like a duck among swans.
A one-woman army attacking the sidewalk with brisk steps
As she marches through jungle of disapproving glances.
I wonder what goes on behind that furrowed brow
And severe stare.
I see a dark face lined with hardships
And wrought with iron will.
I turn up the car's heat as I watch puffs of frost flee her mouth.

The cold wind that swirls around her is muted
By mellow radio, sweet coffee, and locked metal doors.
How many intersections before we really meet?

A green blur becomes apparent and I start up again
Amid a rush of united vehicles.

I sail by, leaving her behind
As we both persevere in our respective worlds.

What if …

What if …
I lived alone in the clouds
High above the rest of the world?
And watched life go on below me
Day in, day out – Watching
Sitting silently on a soft cloud.

What if …
Someone pushed me off that cloud
And I fell down to land amid the rushing world?
Lost among the people, the happiness, the problems, the action
Lost for where to go, what to do, when to do it,
*   who to approach, how to act …*
Lost and stranded.

What if …
I leapt down to a lower cloud – closer to it all?
But still up here.
Now in the company of the highest birds,
Calm, cool, less crisp.
A different kind of soothing.

What if …
I floated further down, slowly but surely
With the birds at my back and the wind beneath our wings?
Passing a few airplanes;
Powerful, complex, sturdy birds themselves.

What if …
I reached out to a plane and accepted a parachute
And soared gently to the earth
And placed my feet on the ground

And kept them moving
And never looked back?

What if …
I walked through the world
With the individuality of a loner in the clouds,
The passion and companionship of a bird, wild and free
And the confidence, comfort, will and belonging of a regular earthling?

Blocked

Silent Snail
Buried in the sharp sand.
Digging an escape
Which constantly caves back in
A world of other creatures –
Mother Nature's team of experts
Surround the Snail's hard shell,
Never allowed inside.
A poke of its head
Is as close as they get.
The Snail watches and waits.
Sees, hears, feels,
But can't change or control them
So pokes its head back in.

Thanks

Wednesday February 9th arrived,
Barely a person, hardly alive.
20 weeks later, here I go
With more than 15 kilos to show.
Without your understanding, guidance & care
I would still be way back there.
I've come only so far & there's much further yet
But my experience here I will never forget.

Finally, it got past the food to how I felt
Now I gratefully carry the tools under my belt.
Your tremendous efforts, great and small
Are so appreciated, I THANK YOU ALL.

Margaret became an avid poetry writer during the course of her admission, and even started entering poetry competitions, which she won. I wish her luck in her future endeavours in this area; she will go a long way.

Sometimes, if we just ruminate on one word, we find that we have a lot to say. Sally, an 18-year-old anorexic patient who had had restricting anorexia for four years, chose the word 'SOME' out of my word bag, and wrote the following poem.

Some

Do you want SOME of my dinner?
Can I climb SOME of the stairs?
SOMEbody ISN'T PLAYING FAIR!
I have to take SOME pills.
Will I go to school at SOME point?
I should write SOME letters.
I want to lose SOME weight!

Sometimes, somewhere, doing
Something to somebody . . .
. . . Someone from someplace
does some thing to me
  SOME things hurt
  SOME things hurt more
SOMEONE never hurt me,
  I did it to myself . . .

Poems can be created very simply after choosing a colour that reflects how one's mood is on that day. The name of the colour is written vertically down the page, and an acrostic poem follows, each line starting with a letter of the colour chosen. Here are two different colours, expressing two different sets of sentiments, by two different patients.

Red

Radiant angels are God's children
Every child is a miracle of love and hope
Desire so strong to hold one in my arms

The patient who wrote this poem was very distressed at the possibility that she may not be able to have children, owing to the toll her illness had taken on her, and because of her 'lost years'.

Violet

Very black
I am in distress
Only me can rescue me
Left alone to cry
Every step I take another battle
Too tired to fight

The patient who wrote this poem had had an eating disorder for more than half her life, as well as having been sexually and ritually abused since childhood. Her condition was chronic.

I have a large collection of animal puppets that I use in many ways and for many reasons in my arts therapies groups. They are particularly useful for warm-up activities. And, again, the acrostic poem written from the name of the animal that has been selected by each patient can promote a lot of insight for the patient and therapist into where the patient may be at the starting point of the session.

Here are six acrostic starter poems, produced by members of the same group at the same session. And though certain patients may have chosen the same animal, it is interesting to note how different their poems are. Also, some chose to change the title of their poem, the animal they have chosen only then being evident in the letters at the start of each line. And one patient writes an activity of her animal selection, not mentioning the name of the animal at all in her poem or its title.

Octopus

One and alone. Soloist.
She stands amid a truth
perhaps devastation

Can run but remains she in
one place. Running to success –
happy. Not belonging

To the world she wishes to
succumb – wanting a part,
a space

Only she knows not how to
enter

Put thee a smile
have ye a life

U know one day it shall come

So keep fighting
keep smiling.
Pain never infinite – it must end
and leave room only to joy.

My Feelings

Puffed up is how my body feels
Ugly feelings of myself whirl in my mind
Frustration and
Fright
In my soul
Never-ending struggle

Fly Away

Feeling like flying away
Lost with nowhere to go
Yet there is this place called home.

Always I feel so out of place
When will this pain ever end?
Again I search for somewhere to belong
Yes I'd like to fly fly away.

Slowly, But Surely

Triumph.
Uncertain but willing.
Ready to try.
Teamwork.
Little steps.
Every day is a challenge.

Lion

Let me get through this horrible time in my life.
It will be over one day.
Onward I go with each day, at least it is a step forward.
Never again will I be where I am now.

Turtle

Terrible
Upset
Restless
Totally humiliated
Lost
Emotionally drained

Sometimes the opportunity to just choose a letter from a bag can produce all kinds of responses. The written responses to such a directive, which are included here, were given by seven different patients in the same group.

'U'

Ugly is your stomach
right now which you
must tolerate in order
for you to have a future
of happiness and health

'X'

Xcited I am that I am
almost done. I hope for
a future of happiness and
health

'O'

I chose the letter 'O' because it best represents how I feel and perceive myself and the way others see me. Perfectly round and fat, always eating to be this shape. The outside edges are soft and gentle, but there is an empty space in the middle. Absent and nothing.

'Q'

Quizened, Quizzical, Quarky,
These are all words that I don't
know the meaning of, just
as I don't know what may
happen in my future.
It's all a mystery.

'T'

Troubled as nothing seems to have a rhyme or reason to it in the internal sense. I am very accustomed to that externally and know all too well that I as an individual have very little influence over that except how I respond. That has become not tolerating the intolerable however when one has difficulty tolerating oneself due to the terrific fragmentation within, the external and internal integrate to the point, at times, of overwhelming 'dis-ease'.

'R'

Rainbows
Rainbows soaring high above.
Symbolizing hope for a brighter tomorrow
Things have turned around for me.
I can keep going on.
I see an end in sight
I can eat and get well
Life will begin again
My friends and family are waiting
    to greet me with open arms.
We will soon be together.

'F'

Fat, fatigued, (?), forever, finished, forgotten, forbidden.

I'm fat and fatigued, and wish that I could just crawl into bed and sleep away my life.

This disease that I fight is fatal, yet I feel like I will have it forever. And therefore am finished and forgotten from this forbidden world.

Finally, it can be interesting to offer a written warm-up exercise in two parts. Here is one that I have found to be particularly helpful for eating-disordered patients, as the following five examples demonstrate. They were completed by patients in the same group at the same time. Part one of the exercise is to identify a strong feeling that you are having and to write about it. When that piece of writing has been completed by all in the group, part two is given: to choose a colour to go with the feeling that has been identified, jotting down six points about that colour. The double exercise gives patients and therapist a double opportunity: to stop the exercise after part one or to go on and complete part two as well. The therapist can decide when she sees the responses to part one whether they can be taken further in a structured way, and whether all group members are equally receptive to writing more at that time.

1a. Envy

This is what I feel toward people who lead normal lives. People who go about a daily routine. People who cope with difficulties and hardships in more positive ways than through starvation. I envy those people but I am terrified to be them.

1b. Green

1. Green is my favourite colour

2. I am green with envy of people who lead normal lives

3. Green to me is bright and positive – it will lead me to my recovery

4. Green is strong which is what I strive to be

5. When I am well, the green grass seems even greener

6. The green-eyed selfish monster in me, known as anorexia, still will not give up its strong grasp.

2a. Angry

I feel angry because I did not gain my kilo this week. I'm angry and frustrated mainly with myself because I'm always failing at everything I do. I don't want another calorie increase. I can't tolerate eating anymore. I don't want to do this anymore. I'd prefer to just go home but I know I'll get sick again so, therefore, I'm also angry at this disease and how much it has limited my life.

2b. Bright Red

1. My heart is red

2. Red represents how I feel, angry and frustrated

3. I filled in the empty spaces and outer edges with red

4. Red is one of the centre colours of my piece

5. Red is one of the colours I dislike the most

6. A primary colour is red.

3a. Raging

There is a raging battle fighting within,
Pulling in opposite directions,
Which side will take over and win,
This makes for long reflections.

3b. Red

1. Raging red of anger overpowers my emotions

2. Roses are red
Violets are blue
Feelings that are said
Are tried and true

3. The dangerous red fire attracts me to it

4. Red stands out, red is flashy, red is really racy

5. I am in the red and am trying to get out

6. Risky, REALITY REACHES ROUND RED ROSES.

4a. Spiritual

I was relieved to see this word amidst the sentences that I had written to describe the colour purple as I have been feeling disconnected from that part of myself for some time. This is something that is and has always been intrinsic to me in its many forms. I have never defined it except to feel and know that the diversity of the universe is a wondrous reflection of life-affirming unconditional love.

4b. Purple

1. *Purple, being the result of the colours red and blue, is one of my favourite colours*
2. *Purple can be subtle or bold*
3. *I like the colour purple's versatility*
4. *Even a dab of purple is noticeable and changes the overall effect of the rest of the colours*
5. *Purple is such a spiritual colour to me*
6. *Purple is so much fun.*

5a. Stylish

I would like to become more stylish as I recover from my eating disorder. I want to improve myself in better ways other than being thin.

5b. Orange

Orange stands out
Orange is very bright
Orange is cheery
Orange is flashy
Orange is stylish
It is hard to make creative sentences with the word orange in it!

The poems included here were written by a diverse selection of patients in varying conditions and stages of treatment. However, after reading all these pieces in combination, common themes and concerns are evident: the causes, effects and consequences of suffering from an eating disorder.

Further examples of directives that can be offered using poetry or expressive writing are given in *Therapeutic Art Directives and Resources: Activities and Initiatives for Individuals and Groups* (Makin 1999). Their suitability for use with general populations is also discussed there.

PART II

The Main Course

It should not surprise us that so many are finding unique value in experiential techniques. The fact that eating-disordered patients adopt physical and often complex metaphoric means of expressing their emotional pain suggests the difficulty we are likely to encounter in asking them to articulate the inarticulable. In moving to spatial, kinesthetic, and symbolic expression, we are, in a sense, agreeing to speak the patient's language rather than our own.

(Wooley 1989, p.vii)

CHAPTER 5

Patterns in Eating-Disordered Patients' Art-Making

The literature on art therapy confirms my awareness of how hard art therapists work and how technical and well thought out their practices can be, particularly with eating-disordered patients (see Chapter 3). However, in the Canadian hospital community to which I belonged, I was often caused to feel I was *just* an art therapist and the work that I did was *just* art therapy. Team members and administrators who have not viewed what happens in the arts therapies group process do not always realize that art therapy is more than arts and crafts. Thus, they are often unaware of the risks attached to the content of artwork, which is confidential as well as serious and sacred. The enlightened support of several mentors and many satisfied patients (some of whose work is included here) are what sowed the seeds for this book.

In this chapter, I set out to show emerging patterns in eating-disordered patients' art-making. Most of the eating-disordered patients that I have seen have been strictly anorexic or bingeing and purging anorexics. Many have been grappling with issues of abuse, either as a precipitator of their illness or concurrently with it. However, no matter where they were in their treatment or recovery, all were mixed together in group, and that group could change from week to week. This mixing was not specific to the arts therapies group, but was the same for all groups and aspects of the in-patient programme. Hence, the materials and directives that I offered were presented in an open-ended way so that all could work individually and to the level of intensity that they needed or could take at the time.

Further explanations of a number of the directives illustrated here, as well as a variety of others, are included in *Therapeutic Art Directives and Resources: Activities and Initiatives for Individuals and Groups* (Makin 1999). Their suitability for use with other populations is also discussed there.

1. Drawing materials

Drawing materials come in so many different forms today. Pencils and markers are not only unicoloured, but changeable, invisible, stampable and blowable. As I noted earlier (in Chapter 3), anorexics are more comfortable with fine pencils, barely making their mark on the page. Bulimics, however, favour thicker markers, and are not afraid of making bold strokes, even extending off and through the page.

Figure 5.1 is a body drawing, very faintly and carefully completed by Clara, a 19-year-old severely anorexic patient who had been ill for three years subsequent to incidents surrounding her father's alcoholism. Another lopsided and awkward body drawing was done by a 24-year-old bulimic and anorexic patient, Stacey, who had been ill for almost ten years and was almost continually hospitalized during that time. The page was torn and crumpled, and the image uneven, cumbersome and disjointed. The pencil marks were so faint that the image could not be reproduced here.

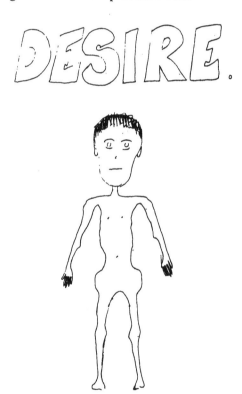

Figure 5.1 Figure drawing, anorexic (Clara, 19, restricting a.n.)

Cathy Malchiodi discusses Golomb's 1990 findings that children may prefer to use a pencil when drawing a person because of the 'complex articulation' involved, and the possibility of erasing any mistakes (Malchiodi 1998). How much should we relate the use of drawing media to the childlike tendencies invoked in eating-disordered patients, as manifested by their conditions? Another observation made by Malchiodi was about how children are influenced by current fads in colour. I note that eating-disordered patients are influenced by all kinds of fads, enthusiastically introducing into sessions the varied array of new art-making materials (such as beads and sparkles) at their own expense. However, the use of these materials is adapted by individuals to conform with self-imposed stylistic limitations directly related to their conditions.

One group of eating-disordered patients that I was working with were anxious to make the art therapy session into a 'fun' crafts group. I wondered whether the essence of the art therapy *modus operandi* might be lost by remaining purely focused on the crafts and shifting the emphasis from process to product. Actually, I had nothing to fear.

The craft activity finally conceded to was T-shirt design using fabric markers. Instead of facilitating an imaginative array of enticing-to-wear designs, the subject matter remained focused on eating-disordered matters. The heavier and easy-to-use markers enabled Paula, a 32-year-old bipolar patient with a 15-year history of restricting anorexia nervosa, to state clearly and proudly where she was now at with her eating disorder, as shown in Figure 5.2. Whether she was able to flaunt her 'wearable art' afterwards I do not know. But, for that moment, in group, fabric markers on a T-shirt made a much bolder statement than regular markers would have done on a flat page.

2. Collage

Collage provides an easy overture into art therapy, particularly for those who have not done it before or are fearful of having to make a perfect product, as so many anorexics are. Flicking through magazines and selecting images or words that jump out can be quite relaxing for bulimics as well, who can gobble their way through stacks of printed matter without restriction. Then, cutting and pasting and arranging words and images on the page offers a whole other set of opportunities for play, reflection and a sense of accomplishment.

Collage can be approached from many angles and for many reasons. For instance, when working in her creative journal, Rebecca, an 18-year-old

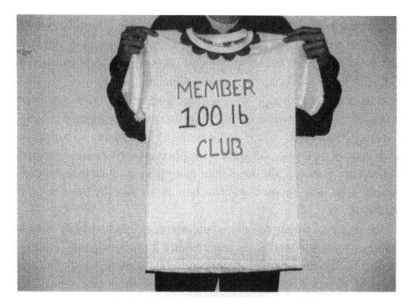

Figure 5.2 T-shirt (Paula, 32, a.n. and bipolar)

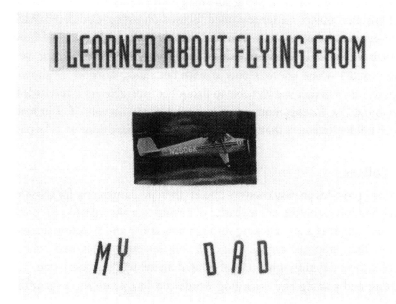

Figure 5.3 Grieving for father (Rebecca, 18, restricting a.n.)

anorexic patient, came to realize, through her spontaneously created imagery, the seriousness of her unresolved grief over the accidental death of her father when she was only eight years old. She had not been the same since. Collages do not have to be complex; Figure 5.3 – 'I Learned About Flying From My Dad' – says it all very simply.

A 21-year-old patient suffering from mild anorexia and more serious bulimia, Janie, created a whole journal dedicated to spontaneous collaging. Janie had also lost her father at an early age, to cancer when she was 11 years old. In her collage journal, Janie went from working on a single page, as shown in Figure 5.4, to spreading her work across two pages, as shown in Figure 5.5. Then, later, she came to integrate collaging with her own drawings. First, as shown in Figure 5.6, she just used pencil; then, as shown in Figure 5.7, she added pastel and smudging techniques. Also, for both of these integrated images, she worked across the double page.

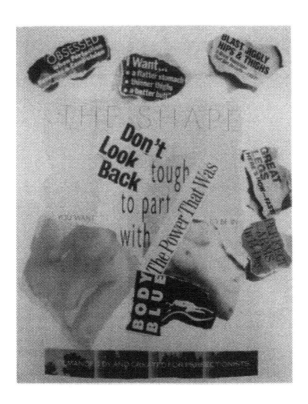

Figure 5.4 Collage on one page (Janie, 21, a.n. and b.n.)

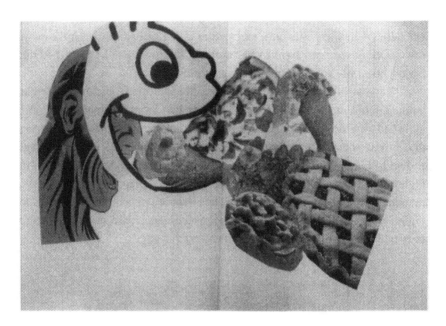

Figure 5.5 Collage spread across two pages (Janie, 21, a.n. and b.n.)

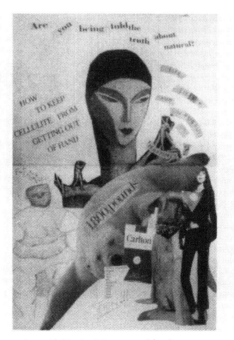

Figure 5.6 Collage and pencil (Janie, 21, a.n. and b.n.)

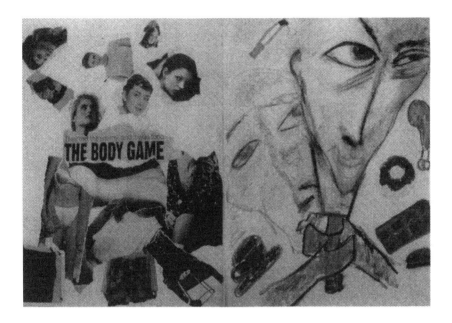

Figure 5.7 Collage and pastel (Janie, 21, a.n. and b.n.)

3. Pastel

Pastels are the middle ground between drawing materials and paint. Yes, fingers do get dirty, but not in the same way as with finger paints. Pastels allow for controlled smudging, and come in two main types: chalks and oils. Chalks, like charcoals, allow for a softer and fainter distribution, with more nuances of colour than oils. Oils require a heavier-handed approach. So, here again, anorexics usually favour the gentler technique.

Due to the range of techniques possible with pastels, they can be used in various ways. Figures 5.8 and 5.9 demonstrate a few of their many uses. These were created by 27-year-old Erica, an overachieving healthcare professional, whose anorexia nervosa gradually worsened over a ten-year period. In Figure 5.8 she is working hard to give up purging activities such as overexercising. This is first shown by softly smudging over her running shoes to haze them out and, later, by making a bold black X, then declaring across the top of the page (with block capitals followed by three exclamation marks) 'GIVE IT UP!!!'.

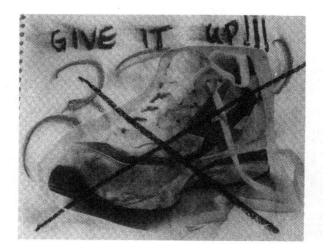

Figure 5.8 Smudged running shoes (Erica, 27, a.n.)

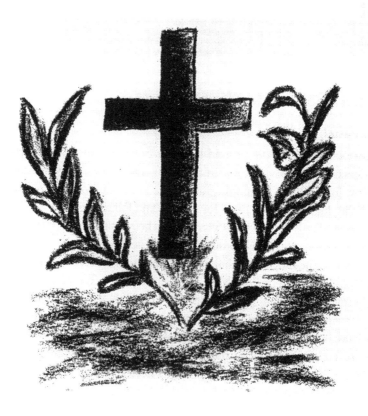

Figure 5.9 Pastel cross (Erica, 27, a.n.)

Also declared in bold, in Figure 5.9, is a large brown oil pastel cross with foliage around it. I have been struck by the number of images concerning both spirituality and death (including graves and tombstones) made by eating-disordered patients at impasse stages of treatment.

Erica also drew two pie charts, which show her trying to focus on making significant lifestyle changes. She divides her time up in two separate pie charts, one from 'before' (her anorexic and bulimic ways) and the second for 'after' (her healthy recovery). The former is smudged around with black; the latter, with yellow. Each is divided into sections that are neatly labelled 'exercise', 'friends', 'family', 'work', 'food', and coloured in shades of green (the shades are so similar that the pie charts cannot be satisfactorily reproduced here). The emphasis changes from 'exercise' and 'work' to 'friends', 'family' and 'work', with 'food' playing a larger role. Since the pie charts and the divisions in them are quite undifferentiated in colour and technique, whether this was intentional or otherwise, from a distance only the externals are markedly different.

Chalk pastels are helpful in enhancing the feeling of a tornado for a 21-year-old anorexic and bulimic patient named Alison, whose condition was triggered by sexual abuse seven years earlier. Here is what she wrote about her tornado, Figure 5.10, after making it:

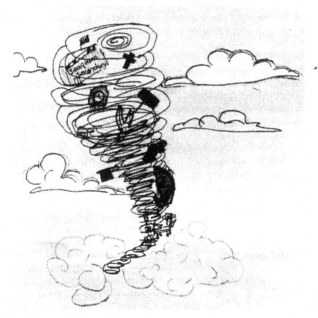

Figure 5.10 Tornado (Alison, 21, a.n., b.n. and abuse)

Issues are whirling around in the space of my head. They are seemingly caught up in a tornado that seems to get bigger and stronger each year as it collects more items along the way, sucking up more and more of whatever is in its path. It is merciless fury that causes me instant panic just to look at it – even the sight of its dusting funnel in the background is threatening. A large part of me is frozen with fear, stuck standing where I watch the huge wind with wide staring eyes and mouth agape. Another part of me wants to rush and bar the doors. However, there is also a part of me that wants to stand my ground, brave the elements, and weather the storm until it may recede again.

4. Paint

Paint comes in many forms, from watercolours, poster paints and acrylics to oils and all types of variants in between. Water-based, faster-drying oils are a marvellous recent invention. However, due to hospital budgets and time and space restrictions, only the more basic media are usually affordable and practical in institutional settings.

Anorexics feel a lot safer applying delicate watercolours with fine brushes to small greetings cards. Bulimics, on the other hand, are fearless, daubing thick layers of tempera paint with heavier brushes on poster-sized paper, not caring if drips fall beyond the edges of the page on the easel frame and floor. Accordingly, while bulimics delight in using finger paints, anorexics find them to be much more of a challenge. However, challenge opens the way for the unexpected. The lack of control felt in being messy causes images to emerge that cannot be planned for in advance.

Figure 5.11 was created by Alison, the 21-year-old anorexic and bulimic patient who drew the chalk pastel tornado (see Figure 5.10); this particular finger painting (Figure 5.11) releases a wave of emotion that leads her to write some powerful associations connected to her sexual abuse:

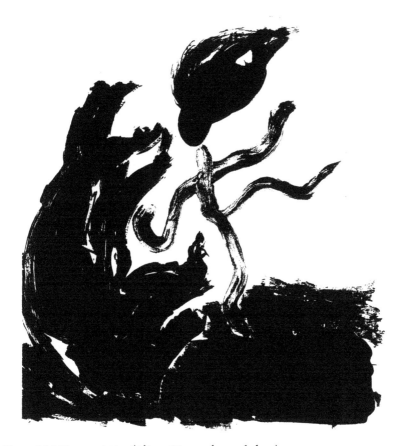

Figure 5.11 Finger painting (Alison, 21, a.n., b.n. and abuse)

Many times my feelings are getting too close for comfort. I want to just flee! Run and not stop or hide somewhere in a dark cave or under the ground away from everyone so I don't have to talk, answer, ask, act, etc. I'm tired of people looking at me. I feel ugly and disgusting. I can't run from those sharp senses any more that terrify me. Smells, touches, sounds, memories, it's very hard to contend with. Like the flames of a roaring wildfire, they grow harsher and hotter as they feed off their surroundings, my feelings of pain and panic or sadness increase as I think about it or something causes me to think about it. This way I'm slowed down enough to feel the feelings; and the fiery feelings grow hotter and more violent as I give them oxygen (by airing them) or feeling them (with memories, etc.).

Alison also experimented with various types of paint, contrasting colours, textures and forms spontaneously, as shown in Figure 5.12. And as images emerged, her experimentation on the page caused her to consider possible new dynamics in her life. She discusses the 'what ifs...' of recovery and relapsing in her written associations that follow:

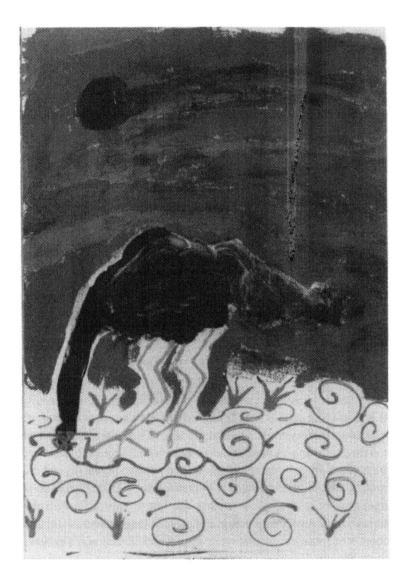

Figure 5.12 Various types of paint (Alison, 21, a.n., b.n. and abuse)

Underneath the surface is a seething, frustrated feeling. I don't know what is causing it: however, I have felt it before as well as the fear and panicky threatened feeling I have been experiencing. I realize I am within a healthier body now. A lot of the time I am scared of these feelings and want to hide. Sometimes my body does tune out and go numb again or dissociate from my thoughts, and actually this can be just as fearful. It is as though my head and body are separating.

Being home and feeling the acute anxiety around food, activity, or other related issues is scaring me into wondering if I will *again* fall into that anxiety and rush of worries that consumes all thought. This has happened each time I recover then relapse and the fear is strong, that I may never rid myself of these feelings. This has increased over time until my fear becomes a panic that hangs over my head and threatens me with bad thoughts. I can sometimes fight it, but this just dulls it and causes headaches as the feelings clash. I blame only myself for all of these obsessive worries. I put them there and remind myself of them so it is my fault they won't go away; why am I so messed up? It terrifies me to think my body will get well but my mind won't. What if my will to get well decreases and the apathy returns?

5. Modelling/3-D materials

Modelling materials, particularly clay, were materials that I had avoided through much of my art therapy training. The dry residue on my hands irritated existing allergies, and I thought it was such a performance and mess, both to get started with and to clean up when finished. I was also strongly aware that I had little talent in using them, since my background was watercolour painting. How different could that be!

Then, one day, I had an important learning experience when we were not given a choice about using clay, and I was forced to come up quickly with a clay product. What an opportunity! I finally had a real excuse to do *real* art therapy, messing up and not making a perfect piece. So, what came out was honest and not contrived, lacking the expertise I knew how to exert on the page that could clip any spontaneity. I not only learned something from my piece and the process of making it, but also about my self-imposed limitations, which I should not have been transferring on to patients.

Because of my own history of discomfort with clay, and since eating-disordered patients usually need to be eased into the art therapy experience, the clay option was one that I initially preferred to introduce later on. However, now, with the wonderful array of safe, clean 'model magic' materials and the like, it is not necessary to wait so long. In fact, the 'clean clays', such as Plasticine, attract anorexics, who tend to model minuscule structures with fine details positioned perfectly – details that my fingers would be too awkward to form. Bulimics, on the other hand, are always ready to slop water on to dry real clay, voraciously moulding larger forms.

Opportunities to work with modelling materials, including clay, make possible the creation of many imaginative structures that can give different impressions and meanings because they are off the page. It is also important to remember that individuals, whether anorexic or bulimic, develop different types of creative expression. According to Lowenfeld and Brittain (1987), the 'visual' and 'haptic' types emerge from about age 12. The visually minded person becomes familiar with her environment primarily through the eyes, whereas a haptic person is primarily concerned with body sensations and subjective experiences felt emotionally. Transferred into art-making preferences, the visual person tends to favour working on the page, whilst the haptic person generally prefers modelling and 3-D experiences. Lowenfeld and Brittain acknowledge that most people have elements of both. However, there are exceptions; I am particularly aware of the significant number of eating-disordered patients who seem to manifest extreme comfort and discomfort with the materials option, regardless of their conditions.

Janie, the 21-year-old anorexic and bulimic patient who had created the collage journal (discussed earlier in this chapter), was also particularly adept at modelling with clay. At the time of her hospital admission, team meetings were held in the mornings. In one art therapy group on the afternoon prior to a team meeting, she made a piece called 'Breakfast, Anyone?' for staff (Figure 5.13). Janie painted the clay to make the food look more real, and was very successful at it. As I have already stated, humour is so important for therapy, and caregivers need humouring as much as patients.

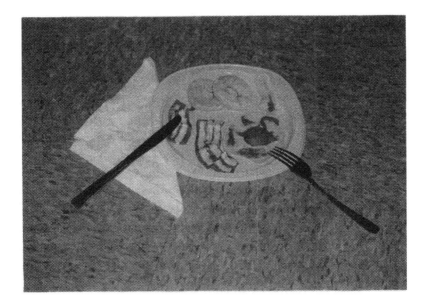

Figure 5.13 'Breakfast, Anyone?' (Janie, 21, a.n. and b.n.)

Using Model Magic, Margaret, the 22-year-old anorexic patient (whose poetry is included in Chapter 4), spontaneously made a simple structure of a head and body. She did this with her eyes closed while listening to music, piling these seemingly simple, but painstakingly executed, perfect blobs one on top of the other, to form a pear shape. The head ended up undersized and the body disproportionately large and undefined. Margaret explained that this figure represented how her body had grown faster than her mind during the course of her recovery. She was worried about being discharged too soon, before she had been able to change some of her thought processes and before she was emotionally prepared.

It has been important for me to encourage and support patients in the use of other forms of 3-D work apart from modelling materials. And recognizing the discomfort that some may have with clay in particular, I often like to follow on from an exclusively modelling session with a variety of imaginative 3-D alternatives. One day, walking home from the hospital, I saw some cheap straw hats in a shop window, and thought about creating the directive: 'What's in your head?' This simple idea proved not only informative, in terms of the creations produced, but was also a lot of fun for patients to do. Stacey, the 24-year-old anorexic and bulimic patient whose awkward pencil figure drawing is described earlier in this chapter, worked particularly well with the hat and related materials, giving new dimensions to the term 'fat', as can be seen in Figure 5.14.

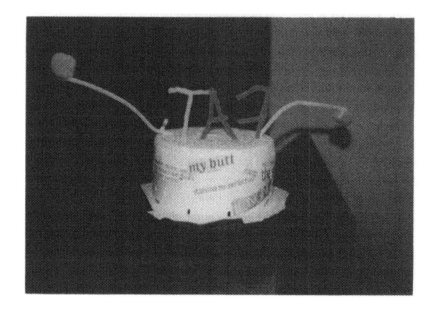

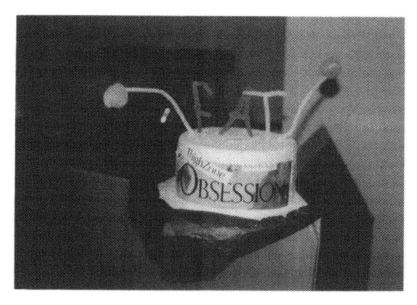

Figure 5.14 'Fat Hat' (Stacey, 24, a.n. and b.n.)

6. Colour

The use of colour is initially quite restricted by anorexics. Everything is black or white. Hence, faint grey pencil is usually their first choice. Then gradually, reds, blues and beiges appear, and not often all at the same time. Bulimics, however, are not afraid to produce bold displays of colour in their very first piece. Malchiodi referred to research by Alschuler and Hattwick that noted that younger children prefer warm colours such as red and orange; older ones preferred blues and greens – the cooler colours. Differences in choice were thought to be due to younger children's natural impulsiveness, and older children's development of a sense of control (Malchiodi 1998). It is interesting to contemplate these findings when considering eating-disordered patients' colour selections.

Lindsay, a 20-year-old restricting anorexic patient who was getting close to discharge, wrote up some reflections on her changing relationship with colour as she started to recover. She named her piece, which follows, 'Uncover My Eyes':

> To an anorexic, life is full of blackness. The present appears bleak and there is nothing promising to look forward to in the future. With the treatment process, as one's body and mind begins to heal, it is as if a heavy fog dissipates allowing the beautiful colours of life to shine through. This enables new, positive thoughts and feelings to permeate the mind of the individual.
>
> Through my experiences as an anorexic, I have been submerged within the blackness. I have just begun to uncover my eyes. To my surprise, I have emerged into a world filled with opportunity and light. As the blackness fades to the background, I see what life is about. There are always tinges of gloom, however the colours which represent optimism dominate my life.

Rachel, a 21-year-old restricting anorexic whose journal entries are included in Chapter 6, expresses similar sentiments.

Crystale, a 25-year-old restricting anorexic, produced two pieces, five days apart, that relayed important information to her about colour. The first was created in her first art therapy group, and the second was her first entry in her creative journal. Though they were in totally different media, the second followed on nicely from the first, explaining and emphasizing for this patient the significance of colour with respect to emotions. Crystale did not give her first piece (Plate 1) a name, but wrote the following about it:

All the different pieces stuck one up on the other represent all my mixed emotions. The shape of the container represents how I seem to be going in a circle, and also signifies the vicious cycle of anorexia. This piece helped me express my emotions.

Her second piece (Plate 2), which Crystale called 'Myriad of Thoughts and Feelings' followed on naturally from the first. She wrote:

While I was sitting outside with my sister and father I felt a multitude of feelings and decided to doodle to relieve stress. I was thinking of when I was younger and looking at the clouds and trying to see figures in them – I feel like my heart and mind are clouds trying to be 'figured out' and full of colourful emotions.

Clara, the 19-year-old anorexic patient whose pencil figure drawing appears earlier in this chapter, illustrates the clear black-and-white thinking patterns of anorexics in her creative journal entry 'Guilty, Sinner' (Plate 3); the meanings of significant colours are explained across the top and bottom of the page: pink for shyness, black to hide behind, red for evil. And in Plate 4, Michelle, a 38-year-old mother of five with a lifelong history of sexual abuse, chronic anorexia and bulimia, and self-harm episodes, in a creative journalling entry puts her arms through stocks, and writes: 'Help. Trapped, bleeding, reaching for the edge. Rescue me. Where is the grey? For me it's either black or white.'

7. Mixed media

Mixed media involves the application of more than one type of art material in one piece. This can be an interesting experience for anorexic and bulimic patients, an opportunity to experiment and mess. For anorexics at their first session, using even one art material can be intimidating enough, but, as self-confidence grows and a need for control diminishes, the way opens to alternatives. Bulimics, on the other hand, often relish the freedom of not having to follow a more restrictive mono-medium format.

Michelle, the 38-year-old anorexic and bulimic patient who put her arms through stocks, created many mixed media pieces, and was the most comfortable when working this way. Figure 5.15 shows two jigsaw pieces from a jigsaw created in an art therapy session, which she stuck into her creative journal. Other patients, such as Janie in her collage journal, have done away with boundaries by working across a double page. But Michelle takes things one stage further by mixing up pieces of sessional work with

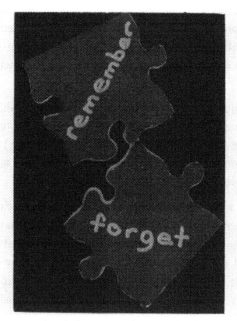

Figure 5.15 Jigsaw pieces (Michelle, 38, a.n., b.n. and abuse)

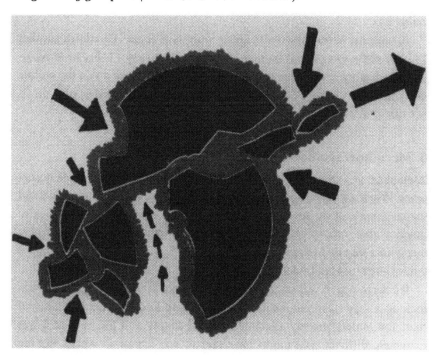

Figure 5.16 Smashed-up CD (Michelle, 38, a.n., b.n. and abuse)

journal entries; everything merges or is merged, literally and figuratively. Figure 5.16 emphasizes Michelle's attachment to recycled materials. She feels unworthy of using anything else, and expresses her pain through a smashed-up CD that is glued on the page and edged with red marker, writing:

> I figure the only way to stop the recording in my head – those anorexic, unhealthful messages – is to smash it to pieces and slowly rebuild one piece at a time. This is a scary process. When I get home I will have no supports, left on my own, but I guess it has always been *me* that rescues me. I wish I could get a prescription for a mom.

Asked to create a 'memories box', the 21-year-old anorexic and bulimic patient Alison encrusted a cardboard box with an enormous range of objects – ribbons, tea-bag wrappers (for dieting), cards and notes of encouragement from friends, and a yellow 'construction' tape such as those used to seal off building sites. She stuck on a big label, which dominated the box: 'The Days Before My Death'. In response to a directive to depict objects of abuse, she attached to a thin wire coat-hanger a pocketless hospital gown that she used to get weighed in, parts of scales for weighing food, calorie lists and a diet cereal box.

In response to the directive to create 'objects of abuse', Charlotte, another 21-year-old anorexic and bulimic patient, constructed a toilet from styrofoam packaging at the same session. She then stuck a ladle down the middle of it (the toilet's basin). This was the actual ladle that she used to stick down her throat in order to vomit.

8. Metaphor/symbol

'Metaphor' is a complicated-sounding word that describes a simple occurrence. When we use everyday speech, it can sometimes be hard to understand the magnitude of situations, and how they might affect others. We may also imagine that others cannot relate to our situations. So, this is where metaphors step in. Metaphor has been around for as long as language, and is a device that aids in understanding.

If I say to you 'It was so difficult; it was as hard as trying to push a ten-ton rock up a very steep mountain', you and I both know the impossibility of that. You understand my dilemma. If I had simply said to you that it was extremely difficult, you might have said to me: 'Okay, so what's the big deal?!' I would then have realized that you could not understand how

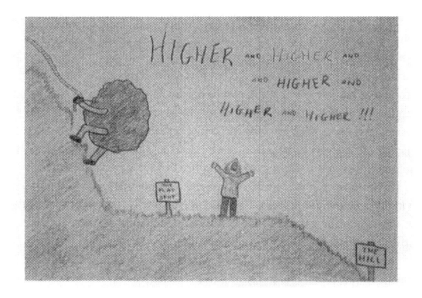

Figure 5.17 Pushing a rock up a mountain (Sally, 18, restricting a.n.)

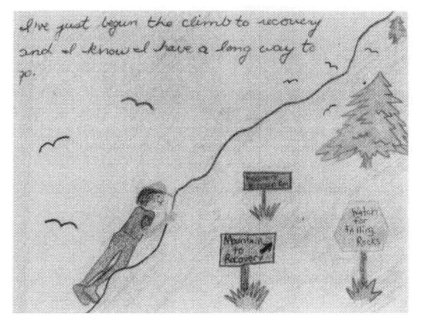

Figure 5.18 Starting to climb a mountain (Rebecca, 18, restricting a.n.)

difficult the task really was. The mountain metaphor is one that appears repeatedly in the artwork of eating-disordered patients with whom I have worked. I include two images here. The first (Figure 5.17) was created by Sally, an 18-year-old anorexic patient who had had restricting anorexia for four years and, being almost due to leave hospital, was close to recovery. In this image, the rock (Sally) is on the last part of the climb, being helped up by a rope that has been dropped down to her for leverage. The second image (Figure 5.18) was created by another 18-year-old restricting anorexic, Rebecca, whose collage grieving the loss of her father is shown earlier in this chapter. Here, she is at the start of her hospital stay, just starting to climb the mountain, but on the right path, taking heed of the signs around her.

The verbal metaphor usually conjures up a strong visual image, as testified to in the previous two images. Thus, art, like poetry, is an excellent modality for displaying the powers of metaphor and facilitating patients' otherwise difficult confessions.

'Symbol' is another word that may require some explanation. A symbol is something that represents something else. When I sign my name, I often add a small open heart next to it. I also use a lot of hearts in my artwork. So I guess you could say that the heart is one of my symbols or signs. Then, if we think about the heart a bit more, and what it might stand for in the wider world, in myths and ancient tales, the reasons why I choose to use hearts as liberally and with the frequency that I do can be explained further. For some, numbers can be symbols, as shown in examples that follow.

'Emotional Numbers' and 'My Fault, My Shame, My Loss, My Pain!' were written by Randy, a 20-year-old anorexic and bulimic male construction worker, whose eating disorder had been exacerbated by a relationship break-up. These are entries from his creative journal in which he spontaneously explores his 'emotional numbers' and grieves the loss of his love.

Emotional Numbers

1 and 2, I feel it,
1 is how I express,
faking #3
causes a lot of stress.

My Fault, My Shame, My Loss, My Pain!

I miss her like a bird missing wings,
   but now it is too late,
So how I feel towards myself
   is nothing but fucking hate.

It was my fault
I can admit
That's why I feel
Like a pile of shit.

He made a series of sketchy images to illustrate and amplify the feelings he expressed in the poems. Directly above the first poem, a stick figure without hands, feet or face, and a head as large as its body, projects thought bubbles in which appear three faces. The first is sad and crying, the second neutral, the third smiling. To the right of the first poem is a face down which tears are pouring, and a wide-open mouth in which is written 'why me????'. To the right of the second poem is a two-tone broken heart pierced by a broken arrow. In the space between the two jagged edges of the break, letters making up the word 'anorexia' are floating.

According to Wood (1996), Levens and Schaverien (referred to in Chapter 3) regard the eating-disordered patient's functioning as being at a pre-symbolic level, her experiences acted out through her relationship with food and her body. The suggestion is given by each of them that the way opens for symbolization possibilities to develop if concretization of experience can be transferred to art materials. Again, according to Wood (1996), Dokter draws on Bion's model of thinking. Through this, she is able to explain how verbal therapies are dependent on the client's capacity to tolerate the gap between the experience of a need and its fulfilment because of the necessity to use thinking (or language) as a bridge. So, it is clear from this that verbal therapies aim at secondary process thinking. Dokter's argument, which is in relation to drama therapy (but extends to other arts therapy modalities), is that 'acting out' therapies, which aim at primary process thinking through the use of symbols for communication, are more appropriate for clients needing to unite mind and body. Laurie Wilson (1985) discusses the work of Beres, who explained that symbolism is one type of mental representation among several, but a crucial one, providing the 'building blocks' for other 'more complex mental representations' such as images, fantasies, thought, concepts, dreams, hallucinations and language.

Not everyone, however, shares the same opinions about the importance of symbolic processing in their work with anorexic patients. Mitchell (1980) has found art-making to be not as valuable for its unconscious symbolic content as for the help it can offer in evoking self-awareness.

As the patient displays her own patterns of experiences and ways of interacting with others through her artwork, she is gradually convinced that she need not function only according to others' mandates. She has her innate ways and capacity for expressing what is going on inside of her. As already discussed (Chapter 3), Levens (1987) insists on the importance of anorexic patients discovering the meaning of their symbolism for themselves. And in art therapy, this is more possible since internal conflicts are projected out on to an external object (the paper or clay), and visual feedback can reflect or mirror that which has been projected or disowned.

Figure 5.19 shows a painting produced by Margaret, the 22-year-old anorexic patient who had made the clay sculpture with a small head and large body mentioned earlier in this chapter. A simple butterfly appeared in many media and forms at various intervals in Margaret's treatment, both in her sessional work (Figure 5.19) and in her creative journal. The drawing in the

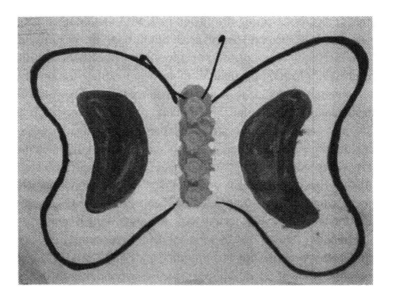

Figure 5.19 Sessional butterfly (Margaret, 22, restricting a.n.)

journal is smaller and executed in pencils and markers. On the lower half of the page is a caterpillar, the numbers 0, 6 and 13 written on its body. An arrow points from the caterpillar to an egg containing the numbers 14, 16 and 18, and another arrow points from this egg to the butterfly, below whose image '21' is written twice. These numbers may represent measurements; however, it is interesting to note that Margaret was 21 at the time of this hospital admission. And at a mid-point in her treatment, Margaret proudly handed me the following poem, written the evening prior to an art therapy session. The butterfly and everything that it represented was impacting her in every language (art and writing) that she was adept at using, giving her, and those working with her, a strong message that she was working hard at recovery.

Metamorphosis

In the beginning ...
a quiet caterpillar crawled.
Crept along with the rest of the world
never quite content.

Took up a hiding place
seven years in a cocoon.

One day a wake-up call
becomes more real with time.
Support from neighbouring creatures
forms the wind beneath new wings.

Shadow of a long lost caterpillar
remains safe and small
within the great expanding wings of a butterfly.

9. Themes

A theme refers to the subject or story on which we are dwelling. Themes can be suggested in group as part of a directive. For instance, I could ask eating-disordered patients to create their ideal or least desirable body images. Hilary, a 25-year-old bulimic patient, spontaneously created a humorous journal entry called 'No One's Perfect Line' (Figure 5.20). In this, she presents an array of individuals all lined up and uttering commentaries about their body images. Other themes that come up for eating-disordered patients, with and without the aid of directives, are those concerning loneliness, isolation, death, hopelessness and suicidal ideation. And depictions of tombstones, food, cages, traps, devils, pets, objects of abuse, toys, perfect and unpleasant settings, intricate doodle designs, masks, isolated individuals and mothers are numerous.

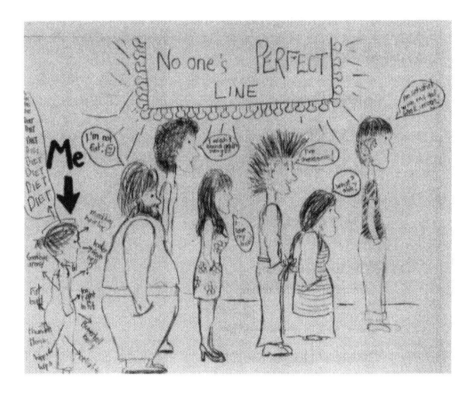

Figure 5.20 'No One's Perfect Line' (Hilary, 25, b.n.)

Twenty-seven-year-old Erica, whose pastel images were discussed earlier in this chapter, drew a picture depicting, with classic anorexic minuscule pencil-writing, a calorie list next to a brain that is spewing out its calculations of them. In another detailed drawing, Erica again applies fine pencil in a classically anorexic way to depict her personal objects of abuse that have aided and abetted her eating disorder: her hands (for measuring and manipulating), belt and ring (for indicating shrinkage), stopwatch (for jogging), calculator (for food calculations), and a cotton thread woven in and around being unravelled from both ends. Unfortunately, both these images are too delicate to be reproduced satisfactorily.

Alison, the 21-year-old anorexic and bulimic patient whose pastel, paint and mixed media imagery can be seen in Figures 5.10–5.12, puts herself in a cage in Figure 5.21, titling the piece 'The Freak', and writing the following:

> I want to run and hide but I am caged like an animal. I'm tired of being analyzed by everyone everywhere I go. I can't just *be*. I must be aware of every action I make or word I voice. I do feel out of control or like I'm on display. I'm a FREAK! Look at me! Look at the FREAK! I'm so disgusting and ugly, people would pay to be shocked by the appearance of such a creature. I can't look anyone in the face when I talk to them myself – consciousness is overwhelming. I fear them judging me – looking at my 'Bucky Beaver' teeth and piglet nose. I want to mame [*sic*] my face – scratch off my nose and break my teeth, pull my hair … LOOK AT THE FREAK!

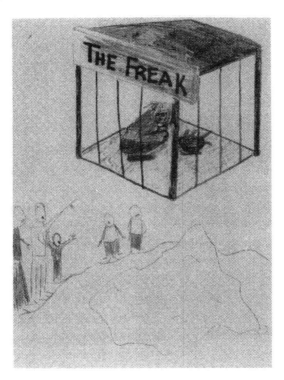

Figure 5.21 'The Freak' (Alison, 21, a.n., b.n. and abuse)

The image in Figure 5.22 was created by 18-year-old anorexic Rebecca, whose father collage and mountain-climbing metaphor picture were featured earlier (Figures 5.3 and 5.18). Here, she depicts an idyllic home setting, full of toys and a Christmas tree, everything perfect and in its place, and coloured in very neatly with pencil crayons. The drawing in Figure 5.23, on a similar theme, was created by 18-year-old anorexic Sally, whose climbing-rock metaphor picture was also discussed earlier (Figure 5.17). Here, she depicts the perfect home scene, with little flowers surrounding a tidy house with a heart on its door, full sun above, and smiling girl next to it. Again, it is neatly coloured in with pencil crayons. Sally also created the intricate doodle in Figure 5.24, which was the first entry in her creative journal, and a faint pencil drawing in which she stands isolated, holding up her mask, while others are happily getting on with their lives together in the background. Sally wrote the following poem about this situation when making her associations:

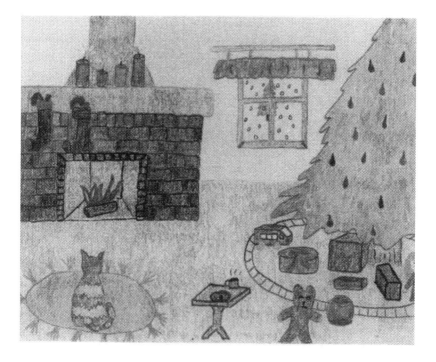

Figure 5.22 Idyllic home, on the inside (Rebecca, 18, restricting a.n.)

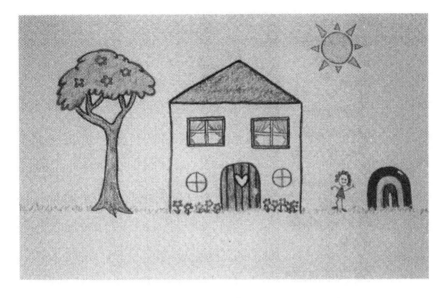

Figure 5.23 Perfect home, from the outside (Sally, 18, restricting a.n.)

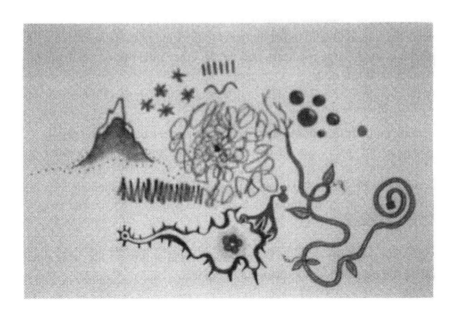

Figure 5.24 Intricate doodle (Sally, 18, restricting a.n.)

My Mask

I wear a mask
to hide my face,
so no one else
can see.

I hide the tears
I hide the pain
I hide the real me.

I don't want them
to see that I
am scared of what
will be.

So I decide to wear
my mask,
until my joy is free.

Also using writing and imagery, Clara, whose anorexic pencil figure and specific colour associations was referred to earlier in this chapter (Plate 3), made a postcard to send to her mother. On the front of it, she coloured with marker a single large red heart, and on the other side, she wrote 'first class postage' and this note:

Dear Mommy,

Take me away from this torture chamber. I have been placed in this prison against my will. I am feeling very alone and isolated. I can't stand watching what others are going through. I just want to lay out in the sun with you beside me. Take me far, far away from this tormented life I am living in. Change my thoughts, comfort me while I don't eat, and you still accept me.

Clara also made an entry in her creative journal at around the same time called 'Death'. This was in the form of a poem:

Death

I want to die
Life isn't worth anything
Pills could be my solution
I am a puppet on a string
I don't want to die
There may be something there
Should I do it anyway?
Why do you even care?

In a group situation, even though patients may be working individually on their own art pieces, when I have asked each person to contribute a line for a group story, more often than not everyone adds similar things. Themes can both unify a session and indicate markers of change, impasses and discords for the whole group or individuals in it. When an individual's themes change, so may she be changing too, whether or not she is conscious of it, and whether or not the whole group is heading in the same direction or at the same pace.

10. Size and space

Size and dissatisfaction with it are central to most eating-disordered conditions. Therefore, when looking at eating-disordered patients' artwork, from size of the paper worked on to where and how images are distributed on the page, certain findings are unsurprising. As anorexics progress in treatment, they feel more and more comfortable with working bigger. Also, bulimics who initially had no sense of boundaries, dribbling paint right off the page, are more able to work within preset limits. Malchiodi, citing Buck, Hammer, Kupitz and Machover, reminds us that most literature on projective drawings points out that the size of a human figure is highly significant, relating it to senses of self-esteem and personal adequacy. Malchiodi also draws attention to other reasons why children may draw themselves small, giving the example of a child whose father was physically abusive to his mother and him. The child, for fear of retaliation, did not want his father to know that he was angry (Malchiodi 1998). Malchiodi comments that when a relationship and trust have been established, figure sizes can change dramatically, even in a short time – a principle that I have found to be equally applicable to eating-disordered patients and their artwork.

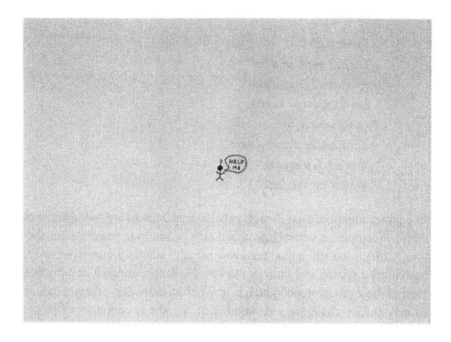

Figure 5.25 'Help Me!' (Sally, 18, restricting a.n.)

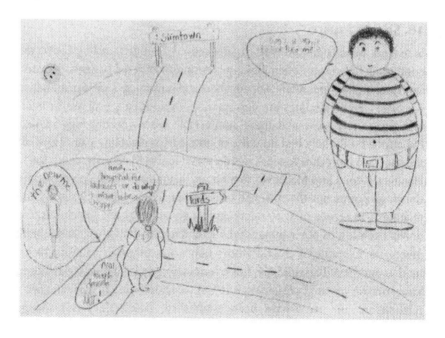

Figure 5.26 'Don't You Want to Look at Me?' (Hilary, 25, b.n.)

I include here two images that are quite representative of the extremes of the anorexic and bulimic conditions. The first (Figure 5.25) was created by the anorexic patient Sally, whose imagery was featured in the previous section on themes (Figures 5.23 and 5.24). Here, she places herself in fine pencil in the middle of the page, so small you can hardly see her or read what she is saying, 'Help Me'. The second (Figure 5.26) was created by the bulimic patient Hilary, whose body image picture also featured in the previous section (Figure 5.20). Here, the page is not big enough for her to work on, so she finds a way to extend off it, by attaching another piece of paper to it, and asks, for all to see, 'Don't You Want to Look at Me?'

11. Charting patterns in art-making

Mary Levens discusses how the anorexic is sometimes frightened of putting anything on paper in case it gets out of control. The bulimic, on the other hand, is often frightened by the strength of her own feelings, which are allowed a 'safe' outlet through art. Bulimics frequently leave little space unoccupied and are often 'envied' by the more restrained anorexics for their ability to express themselves more freely (Levens 1987). Levens also notes that an understanding of the psychopathology of eating-disordered patients emphasizes their immature ego development and lack of ego boundaries. She explains how this is often reflected in their depictions of themselves, giving the example of Lisa, a 20-year-old anorexic patient who had left medical school to seek treatment. Socially isolated, obsessed with her body and extremely unhappy, her drawing of parts of body shapes showed a lack of sense of herself, or anyone else, having a whole body. Levens comments that this is not uncommon in anorexic patients' imagery: 'Many patients with severe eating disorders share common features with borderline patients, in that they are living in a world apart, rather than whole relationships' (Levens 1987, p.3).

In reviewing the hundreds of slides of artwork from the eating-disordered patients that I have worked with over the years, I am struck by how they are when they start their art therapy treatment experience and how they are when they are ready to move on from it. Initially, they are tightly bound up in their eating disorders and related thinking, but by the time their treatment is reaching its conclusion the changes in both imagery and thoughts associated with it are drastically different. Again, here, as in all sections of this book containing artwork, it has been hard to select just a few telling images, that both reflect universal feelings and translate well into black and white reproduction.

Plate 5 shows a creation by the anorexic and bulimic patient Janie, whose collage imagery and breakfast sculpture were featured earlier in this chapter. This was her first piece and she called it 'Body Trap. Will There Ever Be an Escape?' Made out of Plasticine smooshed on to a paper plate, her body is in the centre, chained and helpless, and a snake extends towards her over the red edging of the circle in which she is trapped. I recently met with Janie and her new baby; she has moved on from her eating disorder in that she has been able to complete school, start a career, get married and have a baby. However, she is still constantly mindful of the journey that she has made, and admits to 'lapses' from time to time. Nevertheless, she is careful to not let these get the better of her, especially since her baby is now her main priority.

Figure 5.27 shows a work by Margaret, the anorexic patient who produced the body sculpture and butterfly metaphor pieces discussed earlier in this chapter. This was her final entry in her creative journal before her discharge from the hospital programme. Here, she considers the 'moody gardens' that need to be tended for recovery. By means of a watering can's sprinkles, she is able to review all the elements involved in getting her to this stage of recovery: discovery, independence, friendship, family, esteem, reaching out, emotions, 'nineteen weeks' (the length of her admission), truth, new opportunities and 'why weight?' (the eternal question that needs to be kept in perspective).

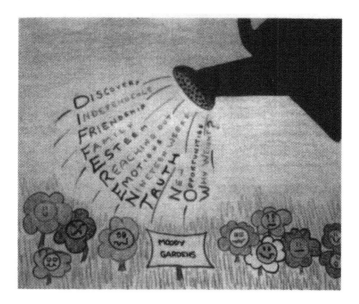

Figure 5.27 'Moody Gardens' (Margaret, 22, restricting a.n.)

I have also found that whatever is depicted in one medium can easily be translated to another; whatever and however someone is feeling will come up over and again in whichever medium they are working until they are ready to move on from it. So, here it is useful to compare Figure 5.28 with Plate 6. They show creations by Michelle, the anorexic and bulimic patient whose mixed media imagery is prominent earlier in this chapter. Michelle starts by creating the initial image of the 'magic wand' in her creative journal (Figure 5.28); then, in a subsequent art therapy session, she brings it to life with pipe cleaners stuck through a plastic glass (Plate 6). Michelle writes about the first image, asking and answering: 'Lost: one magic wand. How do you heal from 30 some odd years of abuse? Still searching and still my heart cries.'

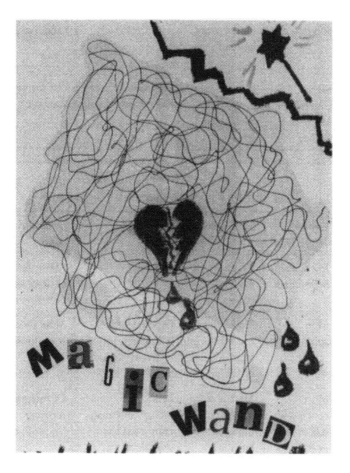

Figure 5.28 Magic wand from creative journal (Michelle, 38, a.n., b.n. and abuse)

12. Eating disorders: Stages of treatment/ recovery with art therapy

Table 5.1 Anorexia nervosa: Stages of treatment/recovery with art therapy				
Stage	Group interaction	Style	Media	Symbols/ themes
I	Isolated	Tight, faint, constrained	Pencils, fine markers, pencil crayons	Solitary people, absence of colour, unpleasant or very pretty
II	More connected	Larger, looser, using more of the page	Experimentation with messier materials, such as finger paints and clay	More diversity and less gloom
III	More concern with others as well as self	More able to make mistakes and mess	Less product-oriented, more process-oriented	Of integration and recovery

Table 5.2 Bulimia nervosa: Stages of treatment/recovery with art therapy				
Stage	Group interaction	Style	Media	Symbols/ themes
I	Invasive, no boundaries	Wastage of materials, chaotic	Paint, clay	Abuse, self-harm, abstract, unpleasant or dramatic
II	More appropriate	Tidier, tighter, less off the page	Experimentation with less expansive materials, such as pencil and marker	More focus and less shock appeal
III	More concern with self as well as others	More able to not make mistakes and a mess	Less process-oriented, more product-oriented	Of integration and recovery

CHAPTER 6

Eating Disorders Seen through Creative Journals

Journalling has become a real turn of the century activity. Many traditional and creative approaches are in vogue. I initiated journalling in the in-patient arts therapies programme in which I worked in the days when I was focusing more exclusively on art therapy based activities. However, as my clinical experience became increasingly intermodal, so did my journalling options and the instructions offered to patients.

Journal-making was one of the most essential parts, if not *the* most essential part, of my in-patient arts therapies group programming. Formal arts therapies sessions took up less than two hours a week, whereas journalling activities could take up as many spare hours in the week as patients wished. I suggested a variety of methodologies that made making journal entries an unthreatening, even enticing, experience. The journal could be picked up day or night; in others' company or alone; when urging to self-harm, binge or purge; or simply for the satisfaction of doodling or playing. Despite the playfulness and humour that can be projected in the pages of the journal, some very serious disclosures and painful episodes can be brought to light in it. Often, it was the journal that provided information for other team members and their groups for the rest of the week after rounds – information about which it was usually hard to talk.

Journalling also provided continuity of care, in formal treatment and for the self. The journal was the ongoing thread and reminder that patients could take home with them as a keepsake and confidant from their hospital admission. Many cannot believe where they came from and to on their treatment journey. Thus, the weekly review of journal images, associations and writings reinforced the verity of their progress and process, and gave confirmational boosts to self-esteem.

1. Journal one: Rachel, a one-time episode

Rachel had had restricting anorexia for about a year at the time of her admission to hospital at the age of 21. Her illness was precipitated by a break-up with a boyfriend, made all the worse by her father's relatively consistent lack of emotional availability and physical absences. Rachel completed her creative journal over four months, approximately the length of her hospital admission. Rachel's journal tells a story that recognizes obvious root causes for her eating disorder. These are processed as and when she is ready; her journalling weaving in, out and around; and reaching healthy clarifications. And during her digressions from her eating disorder itself, there is significant focus on hospitalization. This is shown as an equally traumatic experience for her, producing its own set of symptoms and insights about the treatment system that was as disempowering and disabling as it was helpful.

When writing up her associations to her artwork, Rachel chose consistently to follow the 'Associations Form' format (included in Chapter 9 of this book, and further explained in *Therapeutic Art Directives and Resources: Activities and Initiatives for Individuals and Groups* (Makin 1999)). She gives each piece a name, except in one case where she is significantly unable to find a name. I take extracts from her narratives for the 13 of her journal images included here.

Her first journal entry relates to 'Mud Puddle of Relaxation' (Plate 7). She wrote:

> I used white and blue – a lot of it – because I found it soothing with a lot of paint on the paper. I wanted it to look smooth and kind of 'goopy', I guess. I left spaces around the edges and things didn't go off the page. It soothed and relaxed me when I was doing it. I wanted it to be really big so I could hop in it myself. It relaxed me when I looked at it because I remember how 'goopy' it was when the paint was wet. I felt like using paint because I wanted to use something soft which didn't have any hard edges and something that could change after being put on paper. I did three, all like this one. It was so relaxing that I didn't want to stop. I was having fun painting absolutely nothing, using no brains at all.
>
> I like this image. It was more satisfying painting it, but it still relaxes me when I remember the feeling I got when doing it. I feel as though I can look at it a week from now and still be soothed by it. Its texture when wet is what I wish I could stay like.

The second entry in her journal was a drawing of a bicycle locked to a pole outside the hospital. The bicycle was executed in pencil, while the background was drawn in colour and emphasized the natural world – trees, flowers and grass. Like much of the artwork by anorexic patients, it is too faint to reproduce. Rachel called this piece 'Locked Up', and wrote:

> The bike and pole are colorless because that is like the world is when you're sick. But all around me is full of color which I will be a part of when I am better. Things go off the page, the pole for instance.
>
> The bike symbolizes me. It is locked up to the pole, but with that one special key, it can be set free to go wherever it wants and go to far places. Looking at just the bike, it seems lonely, but with the whole picture together, it looks at home and comfortable. It makes me want to find that special key to free myself of my eating disorder, and get on with my life.
>
> It might not tell a story to anyone else because it's just a bike locked to a pole, but it tells a story to me. I used pencil just because I was drawing a picture, and markers are so bright and cheerful, I think. I like this image, because it means something to me, and it makes me determined to beat my disorder and join the rest of the world.

Rachel's next picture concerns the lack of tolerance for vegetarianism in the hospital programme, vegetarianism being seen there by some as a precursor to an eating disorder. Thus, a vegetarian diet was not an option at the time of this patient's admission. (Being a vegetarian myself, I had to be careful about not letting my countertransference get in the way here.) The piece was called 'Ugly Fish' – an outline of a fish with an open mouth and jagged teeth was scribbled over in pen. Rachel wrote:

> No colors because I see it as very ugly and dull. It makes me angry for some reason. I ate that fish for dinner, and ever since then, all I can picture is a mean ugly fish. When I drew it, it made me mad, that's why I scribbled all over it. I used pencil because it's a dull color.
>
> I'm not satisfied with this image! I've always had a fear of fish, and it was so hard to eat it. The whole time I was eating, all I could see was the fish. I hate fish, and I never want to eat it again.

Figure 6.1 shows Rachel's childish delight at discovering and eating new vegetarian options, even if they were not encouraged in the programme. She called this piece 'Mr Banana and Squeaky', and wrote:

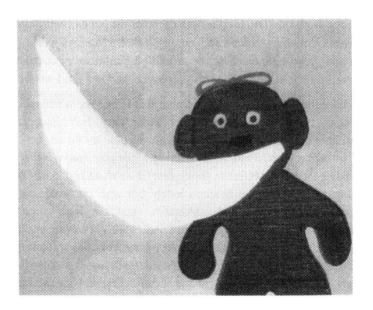

Figure 6.1 'Mr Banana and Squeaky' (Rachel, 21, restricting a.n.)

I first started with yellow because it is bright and makes me feel happy. I liked working big. It makes me smile: yellow makes me happy. When I saw my yellow marker, it reminded me of the peanut butter and banana sandwich I had today for the first time in my life. Once I drew the banana and colored it, it reminded me of squeaky. She's the cutest and she makes me smile. I guess one story could be that my monkey squeaky likes bananas. I used the yellow marker because it is so bright.

I like this image, I think it is more satisfying now than when I was doing it. It makes me smile when I look at it.

Figure 6.2 shows a very product-oriented piece. Rachel discovered a real artistic talent across the course of her art therapy sessions and journalling, which would later be developed outside of the hospital. She called this piece 'Happy Shoes', coloured one shoe purple and one green, and wrote:

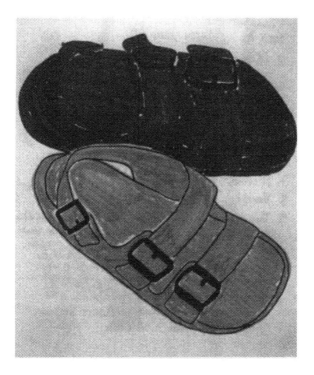

Figure 6.2 'Happy Shoes' (Rachel, 21, restricting a.n.)

I used purple and green which are bright and make my usual brown happy shoes happier. It makes me giggle ... my happy shoes. I could tell a story of guess what!? ... Happy shoes. I looked down, saw my shoes and for some reason they looked as though they had a personality (who knew!). For some reason, I wanted to draw them. They looked so tiny on my bare floor.

I like this image. I find it more satisfying now looking at it. I'm glad I drew it because they're my shoes.

In Figure 6.3, a cartoon character emerges that is later to follow Rachel outside of the hospital to become a trademark of her artwork when she uses it as a model for illustrations in a student newspaper. She called this piece 'Sad and Happy' and wrote:

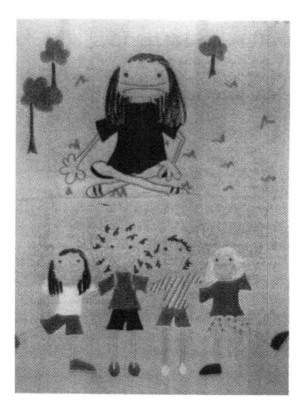

Figure 6.3 'Sad and Happy' (Rachel, 21, restricting a.n.)

I used darker colors on my clothes, because that is when I'm sad. In the second (bottom half of the page), mine and everyone else's clothes are bright because we're happy. The people are me and my family. Each side makes me feel differently. The first makes me sad and alone, the second makes me feel happy and important. I was sad when I drew each because I was drawing myself alone (in the first one) and wanted to be with my family and happy (in the second one).

It tells a story, because while I'm at the hospital, I am alone. There are no close friends, no family, no one with whom I can be myself, and feel completely at ease with. When I am not at the hospital, I can be me. I am happy, and I am with people who I want to spend time with (friends and family). I just wanted to draw what I was feeling, I can't do that with big paint brushes or anything in here. I drew myself sad first because that is what I'm feeling now. I drew myself happy second because that is what I look forward to when I go home at night and when I leave for weekends.

This picture just makes me sadder because I want to be in the second picture right now. It also makes me sad because I am actually alone right now, so the first picture seems *very very* real at the moment. Sitting outside by myself drawing a picture of me by myself, in a sense it is a self-portrait.

Figure 6.4 shows how the journal is handy to have around for difficult moments, when there is nothing else to turn to. The piece is called 'I Can't Sleep'. Rachel wrote:

I used black because it's dark in my room. I'm in the picture and there are a lot of black spots. I makes me feel lonely in a situation that I don't want to be in, when I see it. These are the same feelings as I had while I was making it. It tells a story of me not being able to sleep and unhappy about that and the situation that I'm in.

I don't really like it because I feel like all my nights here will be like this. I find it more satisfying (if that's what you want to call it) looking at it. Although, satisfying wouldn't be the word I'd use. It makes me realize more things and brings more feelings to the surface when I look at it rather than when I drew it.

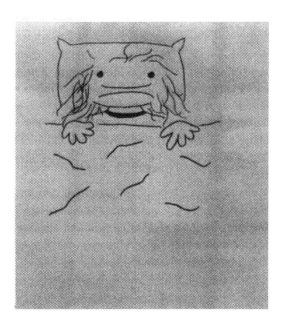

Figure 6.4 'I Can't Sleep' (Rachel, 21, restricting a.n.)

At the mid-point in Rachel's hospital admission, she created 'Distorted', which she has described as one of her most meaningful pieces. A genderless, featureless, faceless outline of a body is faintly washed over with blue, green and red watercolour. Rachel wrote:

> Blue, red and green. I don't know, I guess blue and green because then I think of a 'blurry' color, I think of dark colors. I don't know why the red. I'm in the picture – or my body.
>
> The body symbolizes me, the blurriness around it symbolizes my view of my body – unsure, and hazy, and also not solid (not real). I don't know how it makes me feel – weird I guess. I have no idea what my body really looks like. I know it's thin – I know that, but I guess I don't know how thin. It tells a story in the way that my body is a solid thing, my thoughts though are hazy and not even throughout.
>
> I think looking at it is more satisfying (than making it was) because when I look at it it makes me 'see' that my thinking is distorted and brings me back to reality.

Rachel wrote about a delicate pencil self-portrait which she entitled 'Becoming Myself':

> No colors because I don't feel anything definite: things are still hazy for me. I'm in the picture (it's supposed to be me).
>
> Even though it doesn't look like me, it makes me feel like I'm a person. With the weight I'm gaining, I'm feeling more and more 'normal', like a real person. (My body is getting back to its old self, back to the real me.) I looked in the mirror this weekend and saw my body. I saw all the changes which have occurred. Even though I'm not better yet my body is looking more like a 'body' – not something abnormally thin. Although it kind of scared me a bit, it also made me kind of happy – I'm getting back to a body which is normal for me. This causes scared and happy feelings.
>
> I don't like this picture, I think it looks warped and ugly. I'm not concerned about that though. It was a really strange feeling I had when I looked at the mirror. Seeing a body, not a skeleton, a healthier face, plus my bras are fitting. I didn't feel ugly or hating my blah figure like I have for a while. I felt more like a person, more like the 'norm'.
>
> This all sounds warped, I don't know what I'm trying to say. I guess that even though it raises a lot of scared and nervous feelings, it also gave me happy feelings. I felt more attractive in a way I guess – if that makes

sense. I know I still have a while to go until I reach 'maintenance', maybe that's where some of the scared feelings come in.

After looking over the other [earlier] journal entries, I guess my feelings somewhat relate to questions in the bike picture [see p.127]. I think I am starting to become part of the 'colored' world, and am not as alone and gray. I'm starting to join the rest of the world. I think this is where my happy feelings are coming from.

Rachel comes back to considering aspects of the treatment programme itself, and the limitations of hospitalization, with a picture called 'Hellish Nurses' (Plate 8). She wrote:

It's pretty evident, there's a person. I liked working big. The person goes off the page, and there are blank areas. It makes me laugh when I look at it, it also makes me feel badly because of what I have drawn. I was mad when I was drawing it (obviously).

I think some of the nurses' personalities have a bit to be desired. I'm not saying all of them, but a few. I've really liked my nurse during the past couple of days (that's why orange hair was not included) but some other nurses have been mean to me and made me feel like 'shit'.

I didn't really like working with marker. I feel badly about drawing it, but it helped me relieve some tension where my feelings are concerned with some of the nurses. I just wish some of them would treat me with more respect and I wish some of them weren't so crabby. They make me feel like 'shit' sometimes and about the size of a pea. Some of them are from a place similar to where the red skinned man is from, and I wish I could understand why. Some of them do fit the character of the nurse from 'One flew over the cuckoo's nest'. That's a scary thought!

I still had to show Rachel's journal entries at the team meeting; staff responses were very interesting.

Rachel's subsequent art creations, included here, were key in unravelling what was really going on for her, and to her understanding of some of the reasons for her eating disorder. One (Plate 9) was completed about two-thirds of the way through her treatment; the other (Plate 10) was her final piece. She was unable to give a name to the first, which, as I have already said, is significant in itself, particularly for such an articulate individual. She wrote:

Red and black. Red because hearts are red, and black because the time that has passed lately hasn't been the happiest time in my life – actually it's been the 'poopiest'. Each side of the heart is in it, so I guess that shape is repeated. No people.

I worked small, but wanted to work bigger. I found it kind of restricting. The heart is mine, and it's broken because mine was broken. The two halves are far apart because one is the time when Stuart and I broke up, and the other is now. The black in between shows how the time in between has been troubled and blurred (with a little help from my eating disorder). – That has caused most of the trouble and confusion for myself.

When I look at it I feel somewhat better because there are blank areas on the other side of each heart. Just like there were happy times before I met and went out with Stuart, there are happy times after we broke up. I was sad when I did it. – Maybe not sad, but thinking about things.

I like using paints because nothing is definite, you can do what you want with them. I don't mind this picture. I can't really say which was more satisfying. I guess looking at it afterwards, because I look at it and think.

'More at Ease' (Plate 10) is in direct contrast to Plate 9. Rachel wrote:

Red and blue: red because my heart is red and blue because things are somewhat clearer, or I'm more at ease with things. Also, I liked working this size.

Each side of the heart represents something. One side is the time of grief in my relationship and the other, my life now. The blue is the time in between. It makes me feel better when I look at it and I also felt better while I was making it. I guess it shows how my views and feelings about things have somewhat changed.

I think since Stuart and I have spoken, I've been able to get some of my feelings out and also gotten some answers to some of my questions in my head. This has made things clearer (the change from black to blue, in between the hearts) and brighter. Even though my heart is still broken, I don't feel as hateful (I don't know why) and distant. That's why the two sides are closer, but the side which represents my life now moved back – room for more happiness in the future. – The blank space on the right is bigger, at least I hope it is.

I liked using paints because I found them soothing and not as solid or definite as markers. I like it because it kind of shows a slight change in how I am seeing things or the way I'm feeling. I'm not as sad as I used to be and somewhat mournful, I guess as before. I'm seeing things differently because my feelings have changed. I'm still sad, but not to the same degree.

The illustration shown in Plate 11 was completed a couple of weeks prior to Rachel finishing the programme. It is a very interesting piece for a variety of reasons, from the weight phobia (and number phobia) displayed in it, to the intricacies obvious in the process of making it and the double imagery that both interconnects and jumps off the page with its complexity. It is called 'Fuck', and Rachel wrote:

> They were really the only colours I had. They bothered me though: purple, green and pink. There was no dominating shape and no people. Things do go off the page. I worked pretty big but I wanted to work even bigger. I found the piece of paper limiting. 49.8 is my weight of this morning (fuck!). I don't like the colours. I don't know how it makes me feel. When I was doing it, I was scared, worried and shitting my pants.
>
> This picture shows that I'm now 49.8. The reason why I'm 'shitting bricks' is because now my calories have to go up to 3300. I only gained .3 this weekend (... fuck! ...). I used markers because it's 7:00 in the morning, I'm half asleep and they're the easiest materials to use. I didn't like working with them.
>
> I don't like this picture. I think I found it more satisfying when I was doing it.

Discussing patterns that recur within the different diagnostic groups of eating-disordered patients, Levens describes the anorexic's desperate search for identity through numerous portrayals of herself as different from others. She talks about a 22-year-old anorexic called Martha who did a series of paintings in which she was a different shape, colour or symbol from other people, or separated by a boundary. When making associations, Martha related these depictions to her fears of loss of identity: if she was depicted in the same way as others, she may not be seen by them and so not exist (Levens 1987). It would be interesting to compare Martha's and Rachel's artwork and associations.

Rachel benefitted enormously from the art therapy programme. Just prior to discharge, she recorded how it had helped her to see and look back at things, and remember what she was thinking. What became most clear for her was how alone she was, and how distant she felt from everybody, something that had not been part of her personality before.

At her first session, she had been excited because she did not know what to expect, and nervous because other group members had expressed how they didn't like the group, thus making it hard to know what to expect from them too. In her final session, she came to realize that through the art therapy she had come to understand how she felt about her body and was more able to deal with relationships between other people and herself. She also noticed that she had something concrete to relate to when she put things on paper. More than four years later, I understand that Rachel is still recovered.

2. Journal two: Vera, an older patient

Vera was in her early fifties and a grandmother of seven at the time of her admission to hospital. She had been married for over 30 years, and had dieted since her early thirties, after being ill and having gained weight. 'Success' with dieting led her to bulimic practices, and, in total, she lost over 120 pounds in approximately 15 years. This hospital admission was her first.

Talking about her art therapy experience overall, Vera recorded the following, just before discharge:

> When I first started art therapy I was doubtful that it would help me! My first attempt to express myself was about how 'PROUD' I would be when I left the hospital. I learned many things along the way, however. I noticed how many different 'DIRECTIONS' I was going in, and, 'BECAUSE' these were new to me, I needed guidance.
>
> During my journey to self discovery, I learned how in art to express my 'WARMTH' and find what was 'PEACEFUL' to me.
>
> I will remember the most important thing was not only making new friends, but realizing my 'healing process' had begun because not only am I 'PROUD' of what I did, but I did it for me.

Then, looking back through her creative journal almost two years after her hospital admission and 'recovery', she recorded the following reflections about it, for me to share here:

> After the day that my mother came to visit, I realized that I couldn't keep things in my head any longer, and needed to write down what had happened so I could understand it. I did pictures first, then looked at them and wrote down what I felt after. I had to express myself somehow other than by talking to people and I had to sort it out myself.

The journal was good, particularly for when I was upset or angry, and that often happened in between groups. So, I had something to turn to. At first it was hard to even express my feelings. Then, just realizing I was given a way to express these feelings myself started to help to put things in perspective for me.

The process wasn't as important as reflecting on the product afterwards and looking at it from different angles. On the days when I was angry, making the art actually helped calm my anger; looking at it helped explain it. By the end of the journal I came to realize that I was starting to believe in myself because I had come to learn that I could handle things myself with my own reflections, instead of needing to talk to other people.

What was very interesting and unique for me to observe in Vera's creative journalling process was her use of flower imagery, and the inclusion of a variety of dried flowers, pasted on many of the journal pages and integrated into pictures. She used flowers mostly to represent family members, and they were all shapes, sizes and colours. They were displayed in a variety of settings – with rain, sun and clouds; tall, short or obviously growing. Vera claimed to have no artistic talent and no previous art-making experience; so the amount of effort and imaginative techniques that she put into her work were particularly striking and commendable.

Vera highlighted what she recognized as the three most significant pieces in the creative journal, for her, and I include them and her associations about them here. The first two were done on consecutive days; the final one, ten days later, close to the start of her hospital admission. 'Lifeless' (Plate 12), her least favourite piece, highlights where Vera was at the start of her admission, and she gives this description of it:

> I am trying to 'reach' the sun so I can grow to be with my family. To feel so delicate and fragile is scary. I have no leaves today because I do not have control of my fears, and I can't put my feelings before my family. Before each meal I hope the urge to binge/purge will not be there any more. I would give everything I had to lose this urge. But I realize that I must control it because it will never completely go away. I wish I could find comfort in a shower but I can't touch my body.

Vera created 'No control' following a visit by her mother. An aged dried rose, labelled 'me', has been glued on to a grey-green landscape. Over it hover two large dark clouds, labelled 'fear' and 'rejection'. For Vera, this picture marks a 'turning point', which she describes:

She came here. She intruded on my privacy. How dare she. I told her to leave. She makes me feel so cold, buried and afraid to move. So I survive lifeless under the earth. Am I safe and secure under there? No! I am slowly suffocating. Leave me alone and go away!!

'Tiny Flowers' (Figure 6.5) indicates the love and support of her children (whose names were written by the flowers but have been blotted out for reasons of confidentiality). It was reflected on by Vera in a three-verse poem, showing her resolution and resolve to get better:

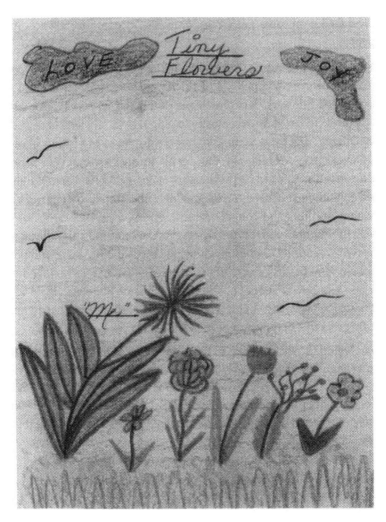

Figure 6.5 'Tiny Flowers' (Vera, early 50s, b.n.)

Together

Time to rise
Time to shine
Time to grow and
   become a vine ...

Invisible me
Lovable you
How can anyone
   protect me so true?

Problems, lies, and fright
Close my eyes, they're out out of sight
This battle is long, but
   with your love I am strong.

Vera also noted that making crafts outside group time occupied her, relaxing her and taking her mind off urges to binge and other harmful activities. These arts activities were also the first activities that nobody else made her do, so she felt free and had a sense of accomplishment.

She also pointed out that when she was first admitted to the programme she was there for her family. Then, after she had completed her first few journal pictures, she realized that she was there for herself. Writing after making imagery and then reviewing both types of journal entry became helpful and enjoyable processes for her.

3. Journal three: Caroline, several episodes and self-harm

Caroline had been ill for about three years at the time of her first admission to the hospital when she was 19. Her restricting anorexia began after her parents' separation, which was due to her father's alcoholism. Once in treatment, it was discovered that she had also been sexually abused on a number of occasions. During her initial admission, she barely spoke and continuously attempted to self-harm. Three admissions later, Caroline has come a long way.

Her third and final admission to the hospital was, at the time of writing, over eight months ago, and I still see her for individual sessions. She is doing well and maintaining her recovery. Very excited about this book, she is anxious to have her personal creative journalling story included, and is currently working on her sixth creative journal. Her story follows, in her own words:

> My art therapy experience has brought me through a long journey. One filled with creative illusions and awesome revelations of an eating disorder. I felt lucky to have had the experience of art as part of my therapy. Without the use of words I was able to express my different moods and attitudes through the simple use of a sketch book and various art media.
>
> My first journal started me on my journey with uneasiness and impatience. My self-esteem being very low, I didn't believe I could create anything worthwhile using any media. The only activity I felt comfortable with was collage. Cutting and pasting was simple and didn't take a whole lot of thought. I felt secure cutting out pictures of skinny models and exercise equipment. These were the types of images I could relate to at the beginning of my admission. Collage really helped me to get my frustrations out and it was quite easy to explain to the group what each picture represented for me at that stage in my recovery.
>
> As far as working in the journal went, my entries consisted mostly of artwork involving difficulties with body image. There was the introduction of the word FAKE which carried through in all my written work. I noticed throughout my first journal there were many entries screaming out my issues, yet in my writing I would constantly deny the fact that I had issues that needed to be talked about. Only now, looking back, can I see the work I was secretly doing.
>
> I tried many different styles of working in the art journal and developed a comfort with writing with the non-dominant hand when I was frustrated (another word that pops up quite often). I introduced my self-harm tendencies into my art journal, sometimes as a coping strategy when my urges were really strong.
>
> The first journal basically consisted of a lot of thoughts without a whole lot of feelings. By the time I was into my second journal, I was halfway through my weight gain and beginning to come alive a little. Facing new issues like exercise urges which took on a life of their own and were expressed through many journalling entries. I began to work on more family issues. Working in the journal helped me sort out and see the difficulties more clearly. The fakeness I was feeling followed me into my second journal along with my continued self-harm.

I remember one of my friends dying during my admission and I had difficulty with feeling anything, so I grabbed my art journal and dedicated a couple of pages to my lost friend which helped me to feel less heartless, especially because of my feelings about death and wanting to die. I used the journal to write about my envy over the death of my friend and the feelings that it should have been me. Feelings that were difficult and embarrassing to express in words.

One constant in my life was the fact that things were constantly changing and my art journal took the brunt of all of my frustrations, changes in living situations, friends moving on (including anorexia, probably one of the worst for an anorexic). I was glad to have my art journal on hand towards the end of my second admission. I was a smorgasbord of conflicting issues and constantly grappling with all kinds of feelings and desires. I was still dealing with all of my anorexic urges (e.g. restricting food and exercising).

When I finally reached my goal weight and received little response from important people in my life, I was having a difficult time expressing everything I was feeling, so many of my thoughts were transferred into artwork and writing. My constant craving for the anorexia; the competition I was feeling with group members; and dealing with the fact that I would soon be leaving the haven I had made my home. I was relapsing before I left the hospital floor, carrying my journal along for the journey.

My third journal began with another admission into a symptom interruption bed. I used my journal very mechanically trying to sort out what went wrong in my last admission. At this point I was doing a lot of writing. All I wanted to do during my brief stay for symptom inter-ruption was to lose weight. So, it was finally decided that another admission would be necessary and I was sent home to wait.

While at home I was consumed with my body and feeling fat, and my art journal was really neglected. On occasion when I had very strong feelings I would turn to my art journal and do a couple of entries. I was almost too numb to even bother, and one entry during this time was just blue paint smeared on a page showing how depressed I was at the time.

By the beginning of my third admission I began feeling really FAT (surprise) and also quite angry. The word frustration appeared again along with the usual self-harm urges. I tried to do something in my journal that showed how much I appreciated the people in the prog-ramme. It felt good to get off the anorexic cycle and have a piece that showed a little bit fun.

This art journal began leading me to make associations with food. At this point in my journalling I was going through a really difficult time, picking up more and more anorexic behaviours. I began writing a lot. I just felt I could express myself the best through written feelings. In the midst of all the turmoil I was surprised to find myself doing a journal entry called 'Celebration'. Out of the blue, I was glad to use the journal in a positive light. It turned out to be a one time thing. Afterwards, most of my journalling expressed how FAT I felt. I also began to make lists. Writing about the advantages and disadvantages of getting well and even little situations that occurred during my admission. Around this time I noticed a shift in the type of journalling I was doing.

The fourth journal began with food associations and self-harm. While shuffling through various types of urges and behaviours, I made a very special friend and utilized the art journal to help me express my feelings about the relationship. At this point in my admission I began using bright colours with a combination of writing and scribbling. The word FAKE still followed me in my journal. I was still fighting and pushing memories away. Again, towards the end of the fourth journal I am full of conflicting issues and huge changes begin to happen.

I was still having many urges and I really tried to use the journal (more than before) to relay my feelings. For example, I began drawing very vivid pictures of self-harm methods and writing about my troubles in group. Saying goodbye to everyone at the end of my admission was a really difficult time. I used the journal to draw little characters (the staff) as a tribute to everyone involved in my recovery.

I was having such a difficult time leaving with so many self-harm urges that it was suggested I begin a whole separate art journal dedicated to my self-harm behaviours. So, I began journal five. Using very vibrant colours and writing, works like suicide and kill appeared. I drew anything that could be used as a self-harm tool (e.g. pills and knives). There was a lot of scribbling which helped with my frustrations. My last entry in that journal was a desperate cry for help which I came to receive through many supportive people in my life.

My most recent journal, number six, began on a pretty good note. I was using a variety of colours and the entries mostly dealt with the future and where my life is going. This journal is a work in progress. But, looking back, I am amazed about how far I have come. The journalling really shed a lot of insight into the way my life has gone over the past few years. I continue working in the journal as a self-help activity and I think

I will continue using it as my life goes on, and more and more experiences happen.

Overall, through all of my urges and hard core beliefs journalling and many other forms of art therapy have provided a healthy release for many issues and I really had a chance to discover little bits of myself, and it will definitely remain with me in my journey to the future.

Caroline's own writings speak for themselves. The imagery selected from her journalling here focuses on her self-harm issues, particularly her use of her nails in this endeavour. There are three different images. The first two are taken from journalling completed during her first admission; the third, from that during her final admission. I also include a fourth image, not taken from her journals. This is a self-harm piece, also about the use of her nails, made in an art therapy session.

In the first image (not illustrated), Caroline cut off her fingernails, taped one to a page in her journal, and wrote:

I had to cut off my nails for the first time in the programme because of self harm urges, and I've already left a few marks on my body which indicated that it was time to take further steps to stop myself. Especially in the state of confusion I am in now.

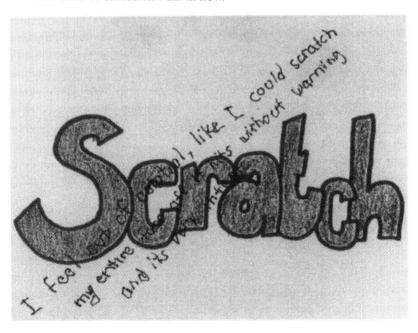

Figure 6.6 'Scratch' (Caroline, 19, restricting a.n., self-harm and abuse)

This marked the first time that she had had to take such a measure in the formal hospital setting, essentially so she would not be asked to leave the programme should she self-harm. Figure 6.6 shows how the word 'scratch' rages loud and clear in her mind – her most prominent thought. Then, once she has got this word down on paper, she turns to her non-dominant hand for a little help in clarifying her thoughts, crafting them diagonally across the word 'scratch': 'I feel out of control, like I could scratch my entire face off. It hits without warning and it's very intense.'

The image in Figure 6.7, produced during a later admission, is a lot bolder than the first two. Gone are the tentative pencil marks and the confusion of the non-dominant handwriting. Now, she is very angry with herself, and scrawls 'Deadly Nails' on top of her firmly pencilled hand in black wax crayon. They jump out at the viewer beyond the page. Her point is made loud and clear, for herself and everyone else.

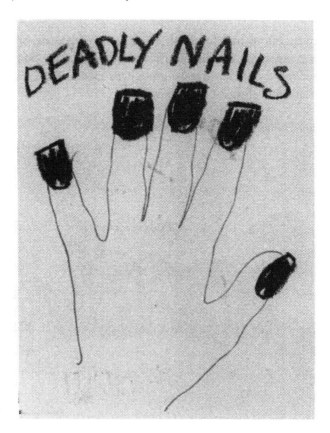

Figure 6.7 'Deadly Nails' (Caroline, 19, restricting a.n., self-harm and abuse)

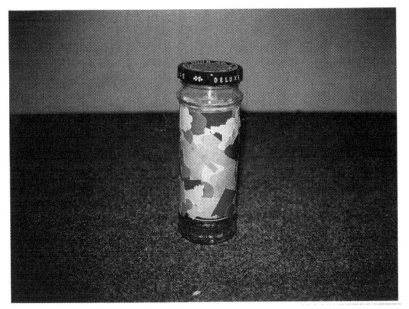

Plate 1 Jar of mixed emotions (Crystale, 25, restricting, a.n.)

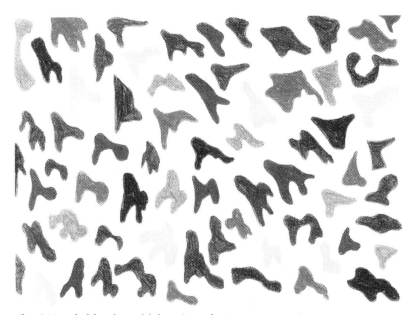

Plate 2 Myriad of thoughts and feelings (Crystale, 25, restricting a.n.)

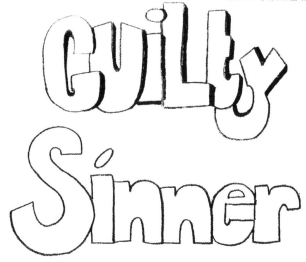

PLACE FOR SAFENESS, PLACE TO HIDE BEHIND. I AM A SINNER. THERE IS SOMETHING TO HIDE.

RED FOR EVIL. SOMETHING BAD. I AM A SINNER. I AM BAD. JUST LOOK BEHIND THE BLACK

Plate 3 Guilty, Sinner (Clara, 19, restricting a.n.)

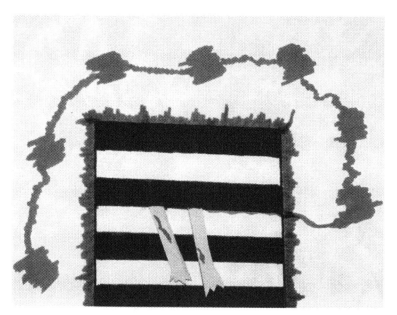

Plate 4 Arms in stocks (Michelle, 38, a.n., b.n. and abuse)

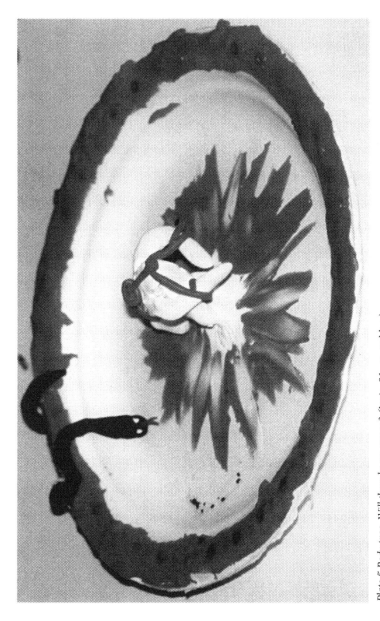

Plate 5 Body trap. Will there be an escape? (Janie, 21, an and b.n.)

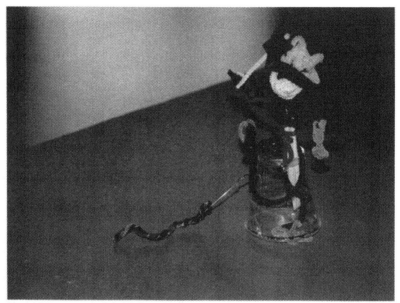

Plate 6 3-D magic wand (Michelle, 38, a.n., b.n. and abuse)

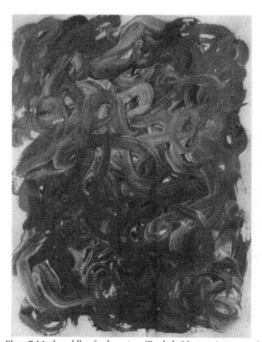

Plate 7 Mud puddle of relaxation (Rachel, 21, restricting a.n.)

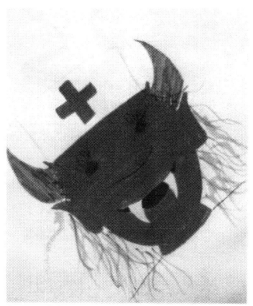

Plate 8 Hellish nurses (Rachel, 21, restricting a.n.)

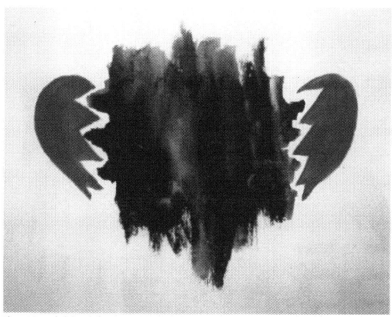

Plate 9 Untitled (Rachel, 21, restricting a.n.)

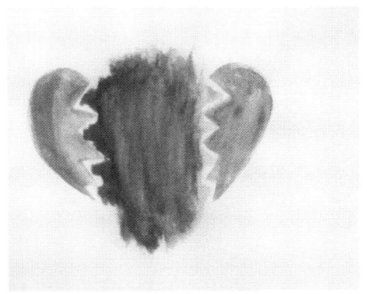

Plate 10 More at ease (Rachel, 21, restricting a.n.)

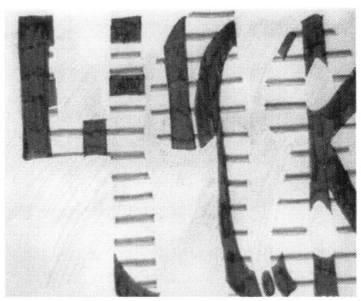

Plate 11 Fuck (Rachel, 21, restricting a.n.)

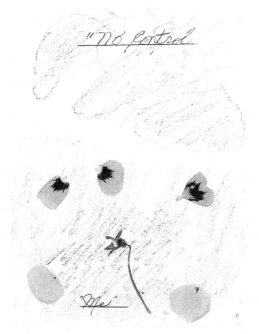

Plate 12 Lifeless (Vera, early 50s, b.n.)

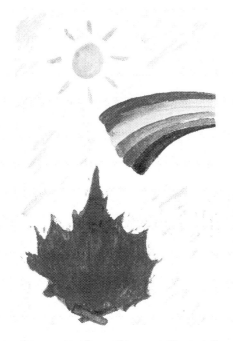

Plate 13 Watercolour flames (Margaret, 22, restricting a.n.)

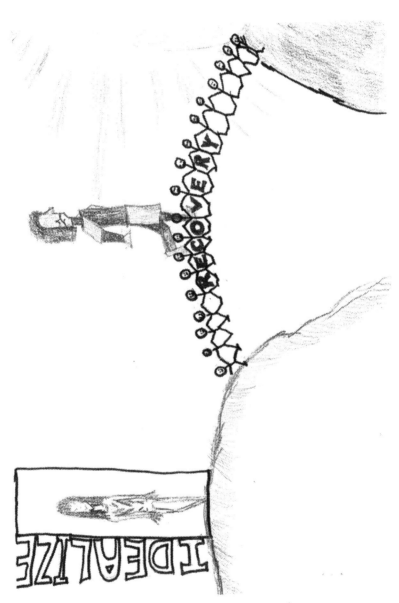

Plate 14 Pencil crayon and marker bridge (Stacy, 24, a.n. and b.n.)

Although the fourth image (Figure 6.8) is not taken from Caroline's art journal, I chose to include it here to emphasize the magnitude of the problem and to demonstrate the patient's willingness to explore it from every angle and in every medium. In the art therapy session in which this piece was made, no directive was given other than encouragement to work spontaneously with clay. Caroline dug her fingernails firmly into the clay from every angle, imagining she was self-harming, and hoping to gain some relief from the very act of so doing, even with clay.

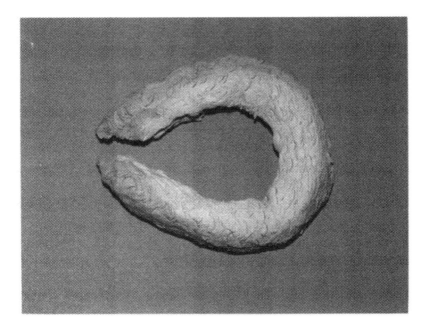

Figure 6.8 'Untitled' (Caroline, 19, restricting a.n., self-harm and abuse)

CHAPTER 7

Intermodal Techniques
with Patients with Eating Disorders

Intermodal work involves the use of several modalities together in one session. 'Modalities' refers to the different expressive arts processes as adapted for therapy. Music, movement, art, poetry, talking or other forms of expression combine to produce a more varied experience for patients. Also, not every patient enjoys or makes progress in every modality. Intermodal work provides opportunities for patients to try activities that they would not necessarily come across in their daily lives, but which can be surprisingly helpful.

I personally recognize the benefits of combining art-making activities with poetry and creative-writing techniques. Because these are within my own areas of expertise and comfort, I find that I have the most skill in administering directives using them. Also, I note that most patients who use these two particular modalities usually have some positive outcome. One modality seems to complement the other; if the visual arts are uncomfortable for an individual, creative writing may not be, and vice versa.

In most sessions, I like to offer a variety of experiences, so as to touch as many of the senses as possible. I think back to my teaching days and what was prescribed to me in teachers' training to make a good lesson. Just as there are different types of learners in school, so there are in therapy. Howard Gardner's *Frames of Mind: The Theory of Multiple Intelligences* (Gardner 1983) is now a classic text, and Daniel Goleman's book *Emotional Intelligence: Why It Can Matter More Than IQ* (Goleman 1995) was a best-seller for many weeks, leading to EQ testing in corporations.

I also realize that in therapy sessions, as in life, all participants are not going to be pleased all of the time; that is just the way it is. At least if they are motivated to be there and can connect with a modality, if not the therapist, shifts can be made.

I have found in 'pure' art therapy that when I offer a variety of art materials there is more chance to engage all group members with something. So, offering a variety of modalities and art materials gives patients more choices. There should be some thing or process that appeals to each patient in some way, so as to provide the opportunity for a meaningful experience on some level, even if it is not an entirely enjoyable one.

Explanations about, and examples of, intermodal directives, beyond those given here, are included in *Therapeutic Art Directives and Resources: Activities and Initiatives for Individuals and Groups* (Makin 1999). Their suitability for use with other populations is also discussed there.

1. With art and poetry

In this section, I give three distinct examples of the use of art and poetry in combination. The patients whose creations I have selected were not in the programme at the same time, and their positions on the recovery continuum, as well as the predisposing factors for their anorexic conditions, were very different.

Marjorie was a 30-year-old with a 15-year history of anorexia nervosa at the time of her admission to the hospital. Her condition had been exacerbated by extreme bouts of over-exercise and flashbacks related to childhood physical and sexual abuse. During a spontaneous art-making session, she drew a picture of a girl, suspended in the air, strings attached to her arms and legs. Above her is visible the lower half of a red, angry face, which may be controlling the strings. She wrote a poem to accompany it, and called both poem and picture 'Puppet on a String'.

Puppet on a String

Out of control
I have no life at all
Just a pile of strings
To lift and let fall

I show no expressions
I would not dare
Don't talk, don't feel
Don't even stare

Out of control . . .
This mouth is mine
You can try your damnedest
But nothing passes this time

Randy, the male anorexic whose poem about numbers is included in Chapter 5, also created a number of significant journal entries using art and poetry. He had never before been interested in writing anything, and certainly not poetry. So, his work in this modality is all the more commendable and significant. He wrote a poem in response to refeeding, which he illustrated with belaboured pencil crayon pictures of the food he described. He calls the poem and artwork illustrating it 'Nightmares in Reality':

Nightmares in Reality

I always thought nightmares
were just bad dreams,
I sit down for snack
and get Boston cream

I sit down at meals
and see blueberry pie,
instead of eating it
I'd rather die

Greasy burger, chocolate donut,
nothing but fat,
it scares the hell out of me
I can guarantee that

I must get better
like I know I can;
I can do it,
but then again,
I'll have to struggle,
and go through pain,
but in the end,
I'll eat and stay sane

Sally, whose rock metaphor and theme imagery are featured earlier in Chapter 5, writes and illustrates a lullaby poem to comfort herself, in her creative journal. The lullaby, called 'Stay Calm', follows here below; the illustration is of a smiling baby in a cradle suspended from a branch. Behind are green hills and a lake full of fish; a path leads directly to a castle on the horizon; the sun is setting and a constellation of coloured hearts watches over the child.

Stay Calm

Calm yourself little one
There's no need to cry
The sun has almost set, my love
The night will soon be here, my love
What's done is done
You can't look back
Hold on to what you have right now
Rest your eyes little one
You've had a busy day

Be gentle with yourself, my sweet
A new day will be, my sweet
I'll hold you tight
You mustn't fret
Life can't be perfect all the time

Pleasant dreams little one
Dwell not upon the past
I understand your fears, my child
I've got hope in my heart, my child
You're not alone
You're almost there
May peace be with you from now on

2. With art and storytelling

Stories can come up in all types of contexts, and even seemingly insignificant objects can be incorporated into an art piece and written about. One directive that I enjoy giving is to ask patients to select a stone from a basket and create a story to go with it. First of all the stone should be placed somewhere in a picture, and then a story can be written about the picture.

Clara, the 19-year-old severely anorexic patient who made the faint pencil drawing of a figure (Figure 5.1), boldly depicted a special place for her stone and excitedly wrote a story about it later during her admission. When interviewed prior to discharge, Clara described this work (the image and story about it) as her favourite from her entire admission. The story was called 'Seeking Tranquility' and follows. I have highlighted some significant phrases in it; they will be discussed at the end of this section.

Seeking Tranquility

> My stone rests on the banks of a cave in Newfoundland. It rests peacefully under a dock where it is washed by the waves. It is surrounded by its rock family but somehow it manages to stick out. Its surroundings are desirable. Anyone would love to live there.
>
> It is a warm sunny day in the beautiful province of Newfoundland. The little town of Seal Cove is bustling with summer fun. Everything is serene, but somewhere around the cove in a quiet little inlet a small little rock washes up on shore. *It seems to disturb the quiet tranquility of the environment.* There is something different about this stone with its unusual grooves and stained colours. Its look definitely tells a story of its long life. *It feels out of place* as the other rocks shift their places, weary of the new visitor to the cave.
>
> Meanwhile, a little girl sits travelling slowly in a little boat, *she feels lost on the waves of the gigantic ocean. She is looking for peace, somewhere to think, away from the bustle* of the town. She finds a little cove, with a tiny cabin and a wharf leading from the ocean. That is it she says. *She has found the place she's been searching for.* She rows up to the dock and settles herself on the way and begins to think. *She feels a bit unsettled, not used to the tranquility and stillness.* She is used to an active life, but *she longs for a place where she can rest.* She begins to feel very alone and as she looks down into the shimmering water she sees a rock but not just any rock. *This rock looks alone and very warm.*

She wonders about the life of the rock. The turmoil of being carried for distances by the huge waves of the ocean. Did it manage to find peace anywhere? She longs to hear its voice. What would it tell her? She decides to disturb the rock's settling place and holds it in her hand. She thought it looked very alone, just as she was feeling somehow, holding the rock.

The voiceless unjudgemental object provided a happy medium. Somehow she had found an in-between. Somewhere between loneliness and overwhelming surroundings. She still keeps the rock with her, and *when she is finding life to be overwhelming and out of control she just holds the rock and remembers the tranquility of the day she found it* and discovered the happy medium in her life.

Stories can be silly as well as serious, and used to engage the whole group with a common objective. In one group session, I had patients each select an animal puppet, then make an art piece in which they created an environment for it to live in, suited to its personality. After each group member had completed her artwork and shared it with the others, I suggested a group story in which each animal came out of its habitat and contributed a line.

One patient took responsibility as scribe and later transferred the story to a computer, making a copy for all contributors and myself. Although there are serious themes behind the story, it is couched in the humour of the more dominant in the group. This story ended up being called 'In Search of Love and Happiness' and follows. Again, I have highlighted some significant phrases in it for discussion at the end of this section.

In Search of Love and Happiness

There was a little monkey named Samantha who was *very confused as to where she would go.* As Samantha was swinging through the trees in a jungle looking for answers, a bright coloured parrot, Albert, accosted her. In the beautiful garden with all the nice flowers, Samantha also saw a bumble bee, Flora, buzz from one flower to another to be nourished. Samantha was *very confused trying to find the right flower that would give her all the nourishment she needed to be happy and safe. After a long time, she found the right spot where she knew she belonged and would be happy and get well.*

From afar, voices of animals were heard. Two approached silently, only their thoughts being heard. 'Ouch,' said the first, Bertha, the donkey, as she noticed Flora, the bumble bee, nipping her on her butt. She was feeling kind of jealous and envious because Flora had found a place of comfort while *she was still lost and searching for her place, for peace and happiness*. And, out of the blue, Flora nipped her again.

She jumped in surprise and ran forward into the worn path in the jungle. And *she ran and ran and ran until she found* the green pasture, which eventually led her to a pond of water, of peace and happiness.

At the pond of water, near the very edge, Bertha heard some very small gasping sounds. Bertha stepped closer to investigate. Concerned, she looked to see the source of the cry. But, alas, there was no one there. Then she heard the sounds again, and, suddenly, saw a little movement near her right hoof. She was amazed that this was the tiniest, greyest, plainest wee mouse she had ever seen. Bertha said, 'Can I help you? *This is the pond of love and happiness and you don't look loved or happy.*'

The little mouse, named Jemima, gasped. 'Thank you. You'll never believe what happened to me on the way to the pond. I was in search of love and happiness when this wild parrot, Alfred, swooped down and took me in his mouth. He flew and flew and dumped me in the jungle. *It's taken me so long to find the pond of love and happiness*. I am so tired but would love to share a drink of the sweet water with you.'

Watching all of these events from a bird's eye view, Patricia, the eagle, *knew that she couldn't solve all of the problems of all of the creatures.* Therefore, *she offered the shadow of her wings to protect them from the sun's burning rays, but not her energy.*

Although these stories were written a couple of years apart, and one was an individual effort and the other that of a group, there are remarkable similarities in content. However jumbled or non-literary the stories may appear to the outside reader, they demonstrate three specific phases:

- *Phase 1*: confusion, tiredness, chaos and aloneness.

- *Phase 2*: searching for a better place; for peace of mind, love and happiness, and all that comes with them.

- *Phase 3*: mindfulness not to take for granted what has been found, knowing how to draw from and hold on to it.

I have found a common message emerging from the scenarios and details of the stories written by the eating-disordered patients with whom I have worked. This is the desire for peace, away from turmoil; the desire for a safe place, where they can feel calm and able to come back to at any time for sanctuary, sustenance, unconditional love and happiness. They are also weary of having to know how to protect themselves, being able to hold on to what they have finally been able to find, and trying to achieve balance in their lives.

Below are the highlighted phrases from each of the two stories, attached to the three phases.

Phrases and phases from 'Seeking Tranquility'

Phase 1:

> It seems to disturb the quiet tranquility of the environment.
> It feels out of place.
> She feels lost on the waves of the gigantic ocean.
> She is looking for peace, somewhere to think, away from the bustle.

Phase 2:

> She has found the place she's been searching for.
> She feels a bit unsettled, not used to the tranquility and stillness.
> She longs for a place where she can rest.
> This rock looks alone and very warm.

Phase 3:

> The voiceless unjudgemental object provided a happy medium.
> Somehow she had found an in-between.
> Somewhere between loneliness and overwhelming surroundings.
> When she is finding life to be overwhelming and out of control she just holds the rock and remembers the tranquility of the day she found it.

Phrases and phases from 'In Search of Love and Happiness'

Phase 1:

> Very confused as to where she would go.
> Very confused trying to find the right flower that would give her all the nourishment she needed to be happy and safe.
> She was still lost and searching for her place, for peace and happiness.

Phase 2:

> *She ran and ran and ran until she found…*
> *After a long time, she found the right spot where she knew she belonged and would*
> *be happy and get well.*
> *This is the pond of love and happiness and you don't look loved or happy.*

Phase 3:

> *It's taken me so long to find the pond of love and happiness.*
> *Knew that she couldn't solve all of the problems of all of the creatures.*
> *She offered the shadow of her wings to protect them from the sun's burning rays, but*
> *not her energy.*

Eating-disordered patients are very often much wiser than their caregivers. They know exactly what they need, their obstacles to obtaining it, and what is required for maintenance of well-being should they recover. Unfortunately, however, life does not always let us identify our needs or provide us with environments to meet and maintain them. Since most research on eating disorders is statistically and scientifically based, I sometimes wonder if fundamental information, of the type that emerges during a standard creative arts exercise, is overlooked. Such information is crucial, both to a full understanding of the patient that is faithful to the complexity and ambiguity of the clinical situation and to an integrated treatment approach. Arts therapies findings could only serve to enhance repeatable and expectable outcome studies.

Regrettably, however, in the professional eating-disorders community, what is considered as 'artsy research' appears inconsistent with medical and psychological models and, despite the resulting insights, is seldom validated by scientific researchers. Then there are those researchers and clinicians from approved conventional settings who work with detachment from the hearts, souls and pains of their patients. It is almost as if some scientists and clinicians are repeating, through their methodology, a fundamental difficulty of many patients with eating disorders – narrowly focusing on one aspect only, not seeing the entire picture, minimizing valuable information. Thus, serious concerns about the increasing numbers of eating-disordered patients with poor treatment outcomes are not surprising.

As so many patient examples illustrate in this book, there is considerable power behind the arts therapies. So, ideally, the three phases listed here, as deduced from the two stories by patients, could be explored further to help in the formulation of successful treatment approaches for eating-disordered patients. These approaches would consider *all* the variables. Quantitators (scientifically oriented clinicians and researchers) and qualitators (creative and heuristic clinicians and researchers) must come together – placing each other's findings in perspective, combining the best of both worlds, and ultimately treating patients more effectively.

CHAPTER 8

Group Work with Patients
with Eating Disorders

Most treatment programmes for eating-disordered patients, both in formal hospital settings and elsewhere, emphasize group work. Schaverien appears to be a lone voice in favouring an individual approach for anorexic patients, stating that anorexia is a very private expression of distress, with control being a significant factor in it. Thus, anorexics may be reticent to engage with others in group, giving 'cheerful false-self presentations'. On the other hand, she notes that bulimic patients often benefit from the relief of being in a group with people with similar difficulties (Schaverien 1994).

I have observed in my own work with anorexic and bulimic patients that once they are engaged in the session, and with their own work, they are seldom bothered by other group members' processes or products. This is also confirmed on their feedback forms. Even if an individual decides to sit off to the side, away from the group, she is still part of it, because the art-making experience, which remains common to all, is not interrupted.

In this chapter I draw attention to three aspects of group art therapy that I find particularly helpful with anorexic and bulimic patients. These are mirroring, sharing and group projects. Explanations about, and examples of, intermodal directives, beyond those given here, are included in *Therapeutic Art Directives and Resources: Activities and Initiatives for Individuals and Groups* (Makin 1999). Their suitability for use with other populations is also discussed there.

1. Mirroring

Mirroring is a key component of group work, and cannot be achieved in one-on-one sessions. In verbal therapy, the imitation and offering of similar verbal communications and physical gestures is significant, but in the arts therapies, where the art process and product make up a large part of the session, opportunities for mirroring are enhanced and increased. Depending on the size and nature of the group and its members, mirroring occurs in several ways, directly and indirectly related to responses to art-making materials, processes and products.

Because of the sometimes infantile behaviours of adult patients with eating disorders, particularly when they are institutionalized, peer pressure and copying can strongly influence the art pieces they produce and the actual creative processes involved in making them. Insecurities and low self-esteem, particularly for newcomers to a group, can cause them to follow others' leads. Then, once on the road to recovery and feeling more confident about their own abilities, their artwork becomes more individualized.

It is interesting to note that at different stages of treatment, different images are created and styles of producing them manifested (see Chapter 5, Section 12). These demonstrate the universal nature of conditions and recovery stages, regardless of mirroring.

Flames and fires are commonly featured in eating-disordered patients' artwork, but they do not always come up for the same reasons. The two examples here are from patients whose imagery has already been discussed in Chapter 5. They are Rebecca, the 18-year-old anorexic patient (who made a collage about the loss of her father, among other pieces), and Margaret, the 22 year-old anorexic patient (who made a clay sculpture of her disproportionate head and body, among other pieces). Rebecca's piece (Figure 8.1) is in pencil crayon, heavily coloured, and was created close to the beginning of her admission when she was very angry. She writes: 'The flames represent the anger I feel towards myself for the feelings I often get. My mind craves exercise, but my body resists the urge.' Margaret's piece, on the other hand, was created close to the end of her admission when she was in recovery mode (Plate 13). This was her first attempt at experimenting with watercolours, and she did not care how her final product looked. The flames reflect the energy firing up inside of her, and the rainbow and sun in her environment. I note here also that on other occasions when, close to discharge time, eating-disordered patients have depicted fires, it has usually been when their periods have come back.

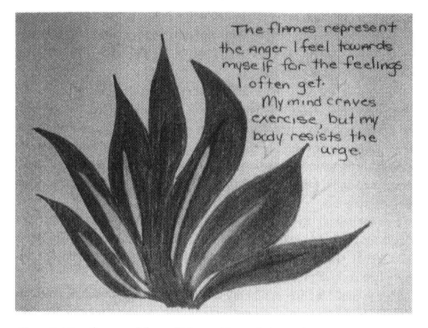

Figure 8.1 Pencil-crayoned flames (Rebecca, 18, restricting a.n.)

Also, when one directive is given to an entire group, it is interesting to note how instructions related to it are carried out and in what ways end products differ. Patients at different points on the recovery continuum are able to work side by side without feeling inadequate, knowing that their creation represents exactly where and how they themselves are supposed to be at that time. The two patients whose art pieces are considered here are Margaret (whose fire image has just been discussed) and Stacey, the 24-year-old anorexic and bulimic patient whose awkward figure drawing, among other pieces, is discussed in Chapter 5. The common directive given to Margaret and Stacey was to create a bridge and put themselves on it, indicating where they were at on their journeys through their eating disorders. Margaret's bridge is a 3-D structure, 'a covered bridge' made from a variety of coloured design papers. Two small stickers, one of a teddy bear, the other of a snake, were stuck at its entrance or exit, each facing different directions. The bridge itself seems solid, but in fact is very fragile. It is a long, safe structure, but it is not clear where Margaret was on it, though the art-making experience itself was a positive one for her, since she enjoyed trying to make something 'different' and having it work out. Stacey's bridge (Plate 14) is depicted in pencil crayon and black marker. It is made up by people who are helping her to recover. She is walking across their held hands, and they are supporting her passage from the idealized body on one cliff side to the sun on the other. She is close to the middle. Stacey wrote:

> The drawing below [Plate 14] is called 'The Bridge to Recovery'. On one side is the sick aspect of my life. The grass is dead symbolizing mortality and depression. The ideal is an emaciated girl; thin, happy, and perfect. Composed of many people joined by their helping hands, the bridge symbolizes the path to a new self. On the side of recovery is life, green grass, and sunshine. I am represented by the purple black person; the blacks representing the mechanical way one must take at times to get better.

Art reviews at the end of treatment are helpful in informing new patients about others' journeys through their disorders, and affirming powerful changes and developments at various stages. I am also interested to hear patients repeat in their reviews, as they do on many occasions, that they were unaffected by others' art-making and products, and able to remain focused on their own.

Not only are art reviews of veteran group members helpful to those who will remain in group after they have left, but the patient who is reviewing her own work notices important progressions, especially if the same directive has been carried out, on several occasions, with distinctly different depictions and results.

One of my favourite pre-prepared exercises is the jigsaw puzzle. I call it pre-prepared because the format is set by the limitations of the card onto which the jigsaw has been punched. However, jigsaw puzzles do come in various sizes, so choices can be made in that regard. Nevertheless, I have found the easiest for patients to work with, usually, is the 8½ in × 11 in piece size. Margaret, whose fire picture and covered bridge have just been mentioned, had the opportunity to create two jigsaw puzzles during her admission; the first close to the beginning, and the second at the end. When she came to do her art review, she was very aware of the stark differences between them. The first in faint pencil was left unfinished, with scratchings of names and feelings, and no direction or focus. The second, in bold marker, was full of names and resolutions, plans, hopes, dreams and wishes. The second piece, in particular, is very specific, reflecting Margaret's clarity and determination on completing the programme. Unfortunately, for reasons of confidentiality, I am unable to show either of these pieces.

2. Sharing

Sharing in arts therapies groups, unlike in verbal therapy groups, happens both formally and informally. Informal opportunities occur during art-making processes, when patients chatter happily and unhappily to each other about their pieces, conditions and beyond. Some arts therapists may discourage 'banter' that the whole group is not privy to hearing. However, in my experience, I have found that as patients assume more relaxed states, once creative processes are underway, they are able to open up in 'free discussion' not directly moderated by the group leader. If talking does reach a level that is disruptive to group members who are not participating in it, interventions do need to be made. But, it should be remembered that the sense of freedom afforded in the art-making environment is very special. Eating disorders programmes are very rigid traditionally; in contrast, the art group's seeming lack of formality allows for more gains than pains overall.

Formal sharings happen during warm-ups and closings, as well as during discussions about art pieces subsequent to art-making processes. During these times, there are opportunities for humour as well as identifications. I am particularly struck by eating-disordered patients' spelling mistakes, which become quite apparent when set out on the table or wall in front of the entire group. There have been many jokes, by both patients and therapists, about possible correlations between eating disorders and spelling difficulties. When the group starts and closes, it is paramount to check with patients how they are feeling. Warm-up techniques such as simple poetry-writing exercises allow for initial sharing to be very concrete since it is on the page. Thus, the different stages and attitudes that patients are coming into the group with can be recorded and disclosed in forthcoming and appropriate ways.

The acrostic poem has a myriad of applications. I have regularly asked patients, on entering the session, to jot one word down (vertically on the page) summing up how they are feeling. Then, taking each letter of that word, a line can be written starting with it to make up a poem. Such poems from six different patients who were in a group together follow. Although some patients came up with the same word to describe how they were feeling, their poems were quite different from each other in content and style. (As I have noted before, conventional therapies too often stop at a patient's initial response, slotting it into a statistical or predetermined outcome compartment, not taking it further to explore what the patient may really be feeling, thinking and doing.)

Confused

*Convinced is how I must feel about
   getting better.*
Often I wonder about my future.
Norman is the name of my dad.
Friends are the most important things in life.
Ugly is how I feel about fat.
Sure of myself is how I must feel.
Education is something I have.
*Dedicated is how I must be to
   keeping my weight on after I leave.*

Blah

Bored.
*Let me be somewhere
   (and someone) fun.*
All fed up. And ashamed.
*Help me be interesting,
   enthusiastic and comfortable
   with myself.*

Sad

*So much pain in this room. So many eyes that have shuttered out the light
of day, hiding in the murky shadows of the mind.*

*A slow death of eternal length. A mind-numbing passage down the
winding plumbing amidst the murky shadows of the mind.*

*Destiny awaits. Please let me help. I cannot bear the solitary confinement
where the stench of human cruelty is rank. Let me be your friend. Let the
murky shadows of the mind release.*

Scared

Slowly moving in an unknown direction
Creeping in a dark forest
Anxious about what will be around the next bend
Relaxing only to catch a breath
Eager to find the way home
Destined to search for happiness among pain

Blaah

Beware, for a cat on her feet always lands, tails never to fling less than high
above ground. Falsely it seems to be dignified and stern. But, it is snob to
the world. Strong within.

Look at the beauty, the glory, the myth. The life of the living, the living of
bliss. Want she the joy, the lost world now found. Earn it and yearn for it.
Look up, never below grounds. For stars shine up high –

Always, eternal, infinite, extreme.

Always of beauty below skin. Pain of remorse of actual growth. The
stronger the legs, the easier the fall. Land on the feet and walk with a tail
held high, always thanking the ground for its presence – The wind dropped
you – but, something was there on which to land and swing that tail high.

Hopeful for the day – which I've reached in midair …

Scared

So scared to remember all that has happened
Can you ever forget 35 years of abuse?
Anxious every day.
Run and hide is my usual response
Every time I think I'm ahead
Down drops another bomb on my wretched life

When a session is coming to its close and patients are invited to share their artwork, it is more difficult for some to discuss their pieces than others, not only because of shyness and lack of self-confidence, but also because of the artwork's content and related disclosures. However, if and when painful revelations are necessitated, the art piece can prove a helpful friend, cushion and translator. Marjorie, the 30-year-old anorexic patient whose 'Puppet on a String' artwork and poem are discussed in Chapter 7, had such an experience.

One day in the art therapy group session, I gave the directive to draw a picture that included three elements: a house, a tree and a person, in whatever medium individuals wished. Marjorie not only worked voraciously with markers on her picture (Figure 8.2) but also on her associations to it, which triggered a series of memories of childhood abuse for her. She called her piece 'An Incident in the Past' and wrote the following about it, which she was able to share with much candour, feeling unthreatened and unjudged in the art room setting:

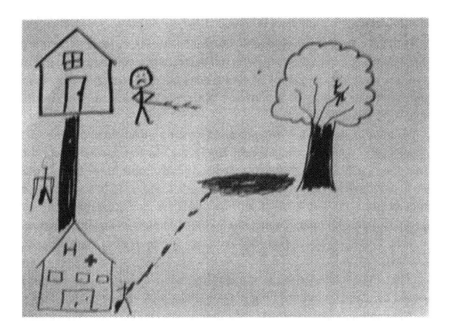

Figure 8.2 A house, a tree and a person (Marjorie, 30, a.n. and abuse)

I used to hide in the trees from my mother. Then, she would come at me with a whip made from tree branches, until I fell out of the tree, in a pool of blood, with broken limbs. Afterwards, I'd go to the hospital and have a cast put on. This was the 'triangle', a cycle that would happen many times.

3. Group projects

The group setting provides both a formal venue for spontaneous individual art-making and an arena for group collaboration on projects. Unfortunately, however, most eating-disordered patients have difficulty combining their efforts on a group page: anorexics are terribly scared of messes; bulimics are not afraid to make one. Product orientation interferes in these circumstances, and patients are challenged on many levels, particularly if they are at different points on the recovery continuum. Also, it is important to keep in mind the medications that individual patients may be on, and how they might influence group performance as well as personal presence.

The relaxed and unobtrusive group atmosphere created when individuals are working independently (on their own pieces) but in the same setting risks disruption when a joint piece is requested. When the group dynamic has the potential of overriding individual needs and interests, issues concerning control and lack of it can easily arise. It is interesting to note how most group projects with diverse groups of eating-disordered patients provide group snapshots that cannot be achieved in other ways, as demonstrated in the following example.

A group project that is recommended for eating-disordered patients in a smaller group (no more than six) is 'The House'. Brown banquet paper the size of a standard dining table forms a handy backdrop with which to work on in paint, markers, crayons or collage materials, and it can be laid down on the floor or a table or stuck up against a wall. On one occasion, when my group had only four patients in it, they worked comfortably together around a table. I shall now describe these patients' house-making processes and products.

First, I was interested to see whether the space (paper backdrop) provided would be used co-operatively or not. Patient A took charge of the project, directing other group members on the initial layout of the house. She worked mostly in her own space, but also went into other patients' spaces. Patient B worked entirely in her own space, which was in the centre of the picture.

Patient C worked in her own space with only a few exceptions. Patient D worked mostly in the centre in her own space, but also made sure she left her mark almost everywhere else.

Second, I was interested to observe interactions between group members, but noticed right away that verbal communications were almost non-existent. Thus, I decided to intervene, and check in with each patient individually to find out what was going on for them. Patient A said: 'Usually, if you're on your own, you know what you have on your mind. This is an "unknown".' Patient B said: 'It's kind of hard because you don't know what anyone else is going to do.' Patient C said: 'I don't like this at all. I feel awkward; but I feel like this anyway!' Patient D said: 'I feel like everyone is doing their own thing. But I'm not worried about what everyone else is doing because it's not being graded.'

Third, I was interested in each group member's contribution to the final product – the house. Patient A, who had taken charge, decided that the house would be depicted in paint, and poured it out for everyone, then said that since there were four of them, the house should be divided into four rooms and each person should take responsibility for one (but there ended up being more than four rooms). Patient A not only painted the black frame for the house (with Patient B), but took care of the land and sky around it, (including a large sun, apple tree and swing), kitchen fixtures and table, bedroom dresser and trees on either side of the front door. Patient B helped Patient A complete the frame of the house and painted Patient D's front door purple. She also put bunk beds and a baseball wall hanging in the bedroom, as well as a deep pink sofa and coffee table in the living room, and dining-room table in the dining room (reworked by Patient D in response to Patient B's insecurities about it). Patient C painted a brown brick chimney with smoke coming out of it into a blue sky with three birds in it. She also added a library in the attic with bookcases, a desk, chair, lamp and large plant. Patient D fed into her obsession with the number five, and put that number on the front door, which she made right away. Then, she added grass around the house and a bathroom with a toilet, bath, washbasin, chair and mirror, as well as putting a television in the living room and reworking Patient B's dining-room table.

Sometimes group projects take longer to complete than individual ones; it all depends on the nature of the project and the personalities of individuals in the group. I am also aware that some patients with eating disorders experience extreme discomfort if they have to focus exclusively on a group piece that is out of their complete control. Therefore, what I have found to be very successful when administering a group project is to allow individual patients to continue working on their own projects simultaneously. This allows for a sense of personal achievement in case the group objective should fail.

Often, when eating-disordered patients are able to divide their time between their own and group pieces, their work on the group piece seems to entail less risk for them. This could be because when patients are not all working on the same piece at the same time, but approaching it individually or with one another, they tend to feel less self-conscious, freer, and more in control of their contributions.

PART III

Dessert

Those who use the arts in working with patients are able to develop people in unexpected ways and to draw out from them the most surprising creative responses... There remains the problem that others may not be converted and there is, unfortunately, still the question of how you get round the problem of the uninterested manager or chairman who thinks it is all a waste of time. In such cases it is a question of 'softly, softly,' of gradually gathering support and stimulating interest amongst those who can be more readily convinced.

(Kaye and Blee 1997, pp.4–6)

CHAPTER 9

Arts Therapies 'How To's' for Eating Disorders

As with other interrelated physical and psychological conditions of varying intensity, there are a myriad ways to work with sufferers of eating disorders. In this chapter, I outline some tips and observations concerning eating-disordered patients, and the use of art therapy by them, as well as providing some model handouts.

1. Tips for therapists

When I started using art therapy with eating-disordered patients, I was thrown in at the deep end. I had no precedent in the hospital in which I was placed; and among local supervisors, expertise in this area was scarce. So as the years went by, I began to make notes about what I wished I had known before beginning. I thought about how I could prepare others, both in terms of conducting themselves with patients with these conditions and with respect to possible limitations and benefits of the art therapy way of working.

The tip list that follows was originally compiled for a local art therapy programme where I have given an annual lecture on eating disorders and art therapy for the last few years:

1. *Be aware of what you wear.* You will be scrutinized by eating-disordered clients as well as other eating disorders therapists. Wearing form-fitting clothes can be a 'risk', depending on your own size and shape, and the transference issues that may be stirred up unnecessarily.

2. *Eating-disordered patients are a creative population,* so let them surprise you with their talents and crafts skills. They don't always need to be instructed on what to do or make, and they come up with some of the best ideas themselves.

3. *Be aware of 'splitting',* especially if you are working on a hospital team. Eating-disordered patients often display adolescent behaviour that commands special handling. It can involve talking behind people's backs; this can be perilous for patients and staff alike who are tempted to collude.

4. *Recognize eating-disordered patients' individuality.* Though patterns will become apparent very quickly, it is important to see beyond those patterns, when and how they come up, and the patient's individual reactions to them, which are not necessarily the same for all.

5. *Know your facts.* Eating-disordered patients are 'authorities'. They may well try to explain to you how they know better for themselves. Also, remember that when individuals are nutritionally starved some of their arguments may lack reason, and their ability to carry out simple instructions may be impaired.

6. *Have concrete facts available for eating-disordered patients,* such as book recommendations. Also, know the eating disorders resources in your own home town (support groups for families, and so on).

7. *Humour is very important.* Don't forget it, especially if the session is very intense. It is not that issues should be minimized; sometimes you and the eating-disordered patients that you are working with just need to take a 'break' from the seriousness of their conditions.

8. *Emphasize the process over the product.* It is important to take pressure away from eating-disordered patients (particularly anorexics) who feel that they have to create perfect pieces. Also, be vigilant about wasting art materials. Some bulimics may get carried away with the quantities that they use. And if artwork is desecrated or thrown in the garbage, it should not be ignored but retrieved for further discussion – concerning both the wish to destroy and discard it, and what it contains.

9. *Consistency is key.* Particularly in groups, the 'teacher's pet' mentality exists. Often, eating-disordered patients vie for attention, and want special exemptions when following directives. The leader may be aware of the varied places the participants are at, and take them into consideration; but making exceptions should be handled with sensitivity.

10. *If you yourself, the art therapist, have a 'food issue'*, you should not be working with this population until you have dealt with it. Otherwise, like unresolved grief, it will interfere with your performance. Try to practise appropriate eating habits and related lifestyle rituals yourself.

Model forms, helpful for therapists' record-keeping, can be found in *Therapeutic Art Directives and Resources*. These are the 'Therapist's Sessional Report' form; 'Arts Therapies Release' form; 'Starting Arts Therapies' form; and 'Ending Arts Therapies' form.

2. Tips for patients

It is extremely important that patients know a little about what to expect from an arts therapies session before starting it. For many, it will be a complete unknown, even the thought of which evokes fear. It is essential that patients, and particularly those with eating disorders, feel that they are going to be in a safe environment where they will not be judged, but will be free to experiment and play with materials that may be unfamiliar but, ultimately, very helpful.

Just prior to their first session or, if that is not possible, at the first session, I usually provide patients with a handout entitled 'Welcome to the Arts Therapies'. It contains two sets of information. Part 1 includes a brief explanation of what the arts therapies are; and Part 2, some recommendations for comfort, during and after therapy sessions using the arts. The text of this handout follows here, and can also be found in *Therapeutic Art Directives and Resources: Activities and Initiatives for Individuals and Groups* (Makin 1999).

'Welcome to the Arts Therapies' handout

PART 1: ABOUT THE ARTS THERAPIES

The arts therapies offer opportunities for creative discoveries and decision-making in a safe, supervised setting. The therapist acts as guide and assistant while the client is free to experiment and play with a variety of materials such as paint, clay, journal and poetry anthology.

Sometimes the art-making process, in itself, can be relaxing and healing. At other times, the finished piece might seem more satisfying to look at or read. Even when something is not consciously on someone's mind, thoughts and desires from the unconscious may surface in the pieces of art that are created. If art pieces happen to take on particular or changing meanings through discussion, the knowledge and insights able to be gained from them are an added bonus.

There are no rules or grades when using the arts for therapy, and prompting by the therapist is gentle. Suggestions for themes to work on are offered by the therapist when necessary, but the client's spontaneous needs are what usually influence the course of a session.

Since the arts therapies allow the client to have significant influence on the direction in a session, difficult subjects may be approached in non-threatening ways and at a comfortable pace. Also, for the 'non-artist', when the risk is taken to use unfamiliar art materials, 'control' is softened, and surprise and a sense of accomplishment often encourage new findings and explanations. The emphasis is not on the beauty or skill and style of the products made, but on the process of making them, and the relief given.

Art therapy involves the use of visual art materials. The client is actively engaged in the art-making process and discussion about it. Art-making exercises tend to be simple and offer variety: cutting and pasting from old magazines, doodling with colour-changing markers, modelling with clean, self-drying clays, and more…

Poetry therapy involves the use of writing and reading materials, such as poetry, journal and story. The client may read and discuss selections already written, as well as being active in the writing process. Writing may come about in response to a specific poem or event or just for the sake of it, whatever wants to come out being put down without worrying about its punctuation or style.

PART 2: RECOMMENDATIONS FOR COMFORT DURING
AND AFTER THERAPY SESSIONS USING THE ARTS

1. Date and number all your artwork, at sessions and in your journal. Keeping records is helpful for understanding patterns, developments and changes that might occur in your life over a period of time.

2. When you get comfortable with one particular material, move on and explore others, maybe even those that you might feel a bit uncomfortable using. For instance, if you like to use markers because they are clean to work with, try finger paints, which can be messy. Sometimes, when you are challenged with unfamiliar or

unpleasant media, what you create might be more meaningful and answer more questions for you, precisely because you are less likely to be able to control it or enjoy the process of using it.

3.   When you have made a number of art products that are similar, think about creating some different ones. For instance, if you always draw houses, you might like to add some additional parts to the picture such as people, animals or a garden. Or, instead, you could start to experiment with modelling materials and reconstruct one of the houses, or make something completely different. The fact that there is a need to repeat making the same art product indicates that it may hold significant meaning. However, sometimes it can be helpful to move on, even temporarily. Creating something new may bring fresh subject matter to the surface that is being denied or connects with the repeated piece and offers supportive insights.

4.   If you are upset or anxious during the art-making process, don't be afraid to speak up to somebody: the arts therapist, other group members, or a friend/family member (if you are at home). The arts therapies facilitate the exploration of difficult and painful matters, but should not be threatening experiences in themselves.

5.   If you are not comfortable with what you have created, think about what changes you could make to the image, object or piece of writing so that it is more satisfying for you. Alternatively, try another medium or scribble freely for a while. This can be done with your eyes shut or with some music that you like in the background, if that will make you feel less controlling or more at ease.

6.   Showing your artwork to trusted others, such as your verbal therapist, a close friend or an understanding family member between arts groups, or when therapy sessions using the arts have ended, may be helpful.

3. Observations

One danger of doing anything for an extended period of time is that we can come to take for granted the peculiarities of the environment. Thus, I have found it very helpful to take as many opportunities as possible to learn from the students and patients with whom I work.

Towards the end of my time working in the in-patient hospital setting, my art therapy student recorded her impressions after three consecutive weekly sessions. Before starting her placement, she had had few expectations about what she would witness, so her accounts were very valuable to both of us.

Session 1

As the eating-disordered patients entered the arts therapies group, their tired eyes, sad faces, and demanding and perfectionistic dispositions were striking. With low frustration tolerances and self-esteem, unpredictable responses, and physically ill countenances, that they were crying out for love was overwhelming. Their bodies seemed to have taken over their minds, or was it their minds that had taken over their bodies?

Once the arts therapies group got underway, however, group members seemed to lift their eating-disordered shrouds, albeit temporarily, and appeared very comfortable, outspoken because they felt they had the permission to express in this setting. It was surprising to see how supportive group members became towards each other. The combination of drawing, writing, and verbalization was very effective in enhancing their communications skills. The art therapist's role as facilitator and supporter of her group members' creativity was significant: they followed her lead yet led their own processes.

Session 2

There was some tension starting this session because the group members did not arrive on time, being held back in the previous group. Then, as both the group leader and group members became more relaxed about situations external to the current group, all were able to start focusing on the here and now.

Most of the group members seemed confused and/or upset when they entered the session, not only because they were late, but because of whatever had happened in the group immediately preceding. By the end of the art therapy group, however, they seemed more clear because of the art therapy process and, more importantly, the art therapist's support. A major transformation was obvious, evident from the smiles on their faces and feelings of accomplishment, which were discussed and affirmed. Prevalent themes arising were loneliness, going home, and mother's crucial role.

Session 3

The group appeared like a family: its cohesiveness was striking. Everyone seemed much calmer than the previous week, especially since the group that they had attended just prior finished on time. Thus, the art therapy process seemed unaffected by other aspects of the programme this time, which enabled it to be more powerful.

That art therapy gives unconditionally (unlike other aspects of hospital treatment) may be the key to its potential for healing, and working on issues of trust, which are crucial with this population. Patients seemed to go from appearing weak, confused, and uncertain at the start of a session to being stronger and clearer by the end of it, in less than two hours.

Prevalent themes arising were shared loneliness, fear of abandonment and needing and longing for mother. No matter the nature of traumas experienced, both being loved and able to trust others appeared essential for eating-disordered patients' recovery.

I also asked patients to consider what their ideal art therapy programme might look like in an in-patient setting. Their suggestions included the following:

1. Two sessions per week of two hours duration each. One session should be spent focusing on art-making in group (new individual and group projects) and the other on creative journalling.

2. The creative journalling session should allow individuals more time for one-on-one supervision. The entire group could work on their own journals, while each person was given the opportunity to have individual guidance, sitting off to the side of the room with the therapist.

3. Less stress on time, because of having a second session in the week for journalling, and formal sessions (with directives) alternating with spontaneous art-making sessions (with no directives).

4. More crafts activities, instead of putting 2-D first (working flat on the page).

5. More instruction on how to use art-making materials and techniques, 'to make us capable of expressing what we want and feeling good about it', particularly where the drawing of bodies and self-portraits are concerned.

6. Optional 'show and tells' by individual patients in group, with
    therapist interventions, to help in the interpretation of confusing
    and ambiguous imagery and symbolism.

4. Patients' associations and note-making

Even when an art therapy group is based more on visual arts, there are still a
significant number of writing opportunities. I have found that even the
patients who are afraid of writing at first, experience little difficulty later. As I
have said before, I think that providing a structure, particularly for eating-
disordered patients, alleviates tensions surrounding activities that are prescribed and would not necessarily have been chosen. It is extremely
important for patients to be able to write about their creations, and there is
usually always something to say. It is just putting it in writing that can be the
challenge. This is for fear of being judged and having to make a written
commitment, which may record something unpleasant that is better not
uttered aloud or shared in any way.

The art therapy jargon for the writing that patients do after creating a
visual arts piece is 'associations'. Associations, briefly stated, are descriptions
or feelings about the artwork created, *what its creator associates with it*. And it is
especially important that eating-disordered patients know that there are a
number of different ways to write up their associations. They should try out a
few of them; by doing this, they will discover one or two with which they are
more comfortable and they will not feel pressured to perform according to
another's mandates.

The methods that patients ultimately choose should be the ones that help
put them most in touch with both their artwork and any meanings in or
behind it, and themselves. A complete list of options follows, but, to start off,
patients may find the first option to be the easiest – just give the artwork a
name or fill in an 'Associations Form' handout. The 'Associations Form'
handout is included after the 'Options for Association-Making' handout.
Both of these handouts can also be found in *Therapeutic Art Directives and
Resources: Activities and Initiatives for Individuals and Groups* (Makin 1999), and
may be used with general populations.

'Options for Association-Making' handout

1. *Starting from a Title or Theme:* This can make things easier, especially if you feel 'blocked'. Or, write about your piece of artwork if you have just made one.

2. *'Stream-of-Consciousness Writing':* There are two stages to this:

   Stage One: Write whatever comes into your head, for up to ten minutes, and without stopping or worrying about punctuation, spelling, handwriting, and so on.

   Stage Two: Underline key words in the passage that you have (just) written, then copy them on to a separate page. The key words or phrases extracted can then be rearranged, either to create a poem or a short prose paragraph, with extra words being added in where necessary.

3. *Non-Dominant Handwriting:* Using the hand that you don't usually write with, write a few sentences about how you are feeling, an object in the room that you are sitting in or a piece of artwork that you may have just created.

4. *A Letter:* Write a letter to or from you, somebody else, an object in the room that you are sitting in or a piece of artwork that you have just created. The letter may discuss a wide range of subjects, from the weather to a sad or happy event that has happened recently.

5. *A Story:* Write a short story about something going on in your life at the moment. You may change some of the characters and their names if that makes you feel more comfortable, or to make the story more interesting.

6. *A Play:* Make up a short play. Use pieces of fruit or animals for characters if you don't want to use people. Also, one of the pieces of fruit or animals could be the narrator (yourself).

7. *A Poem:* Compose a poem about an object in the room that you are sitting in or a piece of artwork that you have just made. It may be written to or from it.

8. *Questions:* Ask an object in the room that you are sitting in or a piece of artwork that you have just created questions.

9. *Answers*: The object or piece of artwork (just questioned) gives answers. These answers may in turn lead you to ask more questions.

As already stated, the 'Associations Form' handout is an easier alternative, where patients simply need to fill in answers to the questions that are appropriate for the artwork that they have created. The form format both encourages briefer answers and prompts ideas. Then, if patients find out that they actually do have more to say about a particular aspect of a piece or the process of making it, they can always choose to continue with one of the other association-making options (from the 'Options for Association-Making' handout).

'Associations Form' handout

In looking at your artwork after you have completed it, you may like to consider the following:

1. *Colours*

    Which colours do you use? How much of them? Why?

2. *Forms*

    Does one type of shape or line come up more often than others? Are there people included?

3. *Texture*

    Is it important for the effect or does it not matter? Is it smooth or rough?

4. *Space*

    Do things go off the page? Are there blank areas? Did you like working big or small?

5. *Symbols*

    Do you have a special sign or number that you have included in the artwork and what does it mean for you?

6. *Mood/affect*

    How does the artwork make you feel when you look at it (the final product)? How did you feel when you were creating it (the process of making it)?

7. *Materials*

   Why did you choose the materials that you did? Did you like using them?

8. *The product*

   Do you like the artwork that you have made? Was the process of making it more satisfying for you (than looking at it is now)? How do you feel about having made it?

9. *Themes*

   Does your artwork tell a story or focus on (a) particular subject(s)?

10. *Sequence*

    If you did make more than one piece of art, do you have any reflections about the order in which you made them?

Also, particularly during a group therapy session, it is important for a patient to be able to reflect on where she is at, and note any changes in mood as the session progresses. Therefore, I include here questions taken from a form for patients to use for those purposes – the 'Patient's Sessional Report'. This is helpful for the patients' charting of their own processes and for therapists to read after the session, to have first-hand accounts documented. It is also included in *Therapeutic Art Directives and Resources: Activities and Initiatives for Individuals and Groups* (Makin 1999).

'Patient's Sessional Report' form

1. Name and location:
2. Date and session number:
3. How are you feeling today?
4. How are you feeling being in this arts therapies session, noting any changes as the session goes on?
5. If you are in a group, how many people are in it, and how are you being affected by other members and their artwork?
6. What is your choice of materials, if you had a choice? Whether you had a choice, or not, were you comfortable with the materials and techniques that you used?

7. Which seems more satisfying, the art-making process or the looking at the product you have made, and why?

8. Talk about what you have created: what is/are the name(s) of your piece(s)? What might it/they mean to you, and how do you feel discussing it/them?

CHAPTER 10

Introducing Creative Journalling

1. About journalling

Journal entries have been a source of much attention for generations, and the contents of many have been turned into best-selling books. These books have been so popular because it is easy to identify with the intricate details of people's daily lives included in them in first person narrative. Whether written at times of crisis, such as *Anne Frank: The Diary of a Young Girl*, or about some of the humorous behaviour of modern life, such as *Bridget Jones's Diary* (by Helen Fielding), the relief that their authors have experienced through writing spills over into our own situations and thoughts, and lets us know that we are not alone.

Journal writing takes on many forms, and there are numerous books and classes outlining specific ways to do it. I have found when working with eating-disordered patients, many of whom are already prolific journal writers, that suggesting options is important; but so too is freedom, and the introduction of ways that are a little different.

Once a journal has been initiated the person keeping it comes to realize its adaptability very quickly. It may be used any time, any place and for any reason, becoming a trusted witness and guide to have available at challenging times. And if sessions with an arts therapist are concurrent, there should be opportunities to receive supervision on journalling work, discussing particular entries and responses to them. So when formal treatment has been terminated, journal-making processes will not only be familiar, but the confidence to check in with oneself when reviewing entries will have been gained.

The journal, it must be remembered, is for the person making entries in it to inform herself, not to impress others; it is to allow whatever is significant for her at the time to exist. There should be no worries about trying to control what to include, but a giving of permission to oneself to let whatever comes out, however and whenever it needs to do so.

2. Focusing on creative journalling

The inclusion of art-making as well as writing in a journal allows for more possibilities. If we cannot be truthful with ourselves in our journal, where can we be? But, often, in 'words-only' journals, the 'system' is known too well, which makes it quite easy for lies to be perpetuated in content. And since deception is a chief characteristic of those with eating disorders, it is important to keep that in mind.

However, when the journaller starts with an image, and allows it to take form spontaneously, and is open to exploring whatever comes up in it, it can be quite an eye-opener. The type of journal that I encourage eating-disordered patients to make I call a 'creative journal', because inside of it anything goes and in any way. The creative journal is a very handy friend to turn to between art therapy groups or other formal parts of residential eating disorders programmes. And, if started during a hospital admission, using it there provides an opportunity to develop 'take-home' skills that will become routine and familiar for the patient for when she returns to her own environment.

The creative journal that I model for eating-disordered patients has a strong emphasis on visual art entries (drawings, doodles, collage, photographs, painting, and so on) and a variety of forms of writing (poetry, prose, storytelling, note-making, and so on), or a combination. Ideally, I advise patients to start with the image and then go on to the writing. Through regular practice with art-making, in particular, patients appear to become more relaxed with materials and techniques as well as experiencing the benefits of the meditative state that process-oriented art-making often produces.

Therapeutic Art Directives and Resources: Activities and Initiatives for Individuals and Groups (Makin 1999) continues from here with information on how to start a creative journal. It includes sample patient handouts, suggestions for subject matter that might be focused on in creative journalling entries, and a creative journalling kit model.

3. Creative journalling and patients with eating disorders

Initially, when I gave out journalling kits, I would let my eating-disordered patients choose from three different sizes of journals: small, medium and large. And, of course, patients chose the size of their journal according to their condition, with anorexics selecting the smallest, and bulimics, the largest. I then thought it would be useful, at least to start off, to present everyone with the same middle ground, a mid-sized journal (7 in × 10 in), as suggested in the creative journalling model kit list in *Therapeutic Art Directives and Resources*.

Nevertheless, even when the standard mid-sized art journals are given out, patients find new ways of using and not using them. Cindy, a 25-year-old restricting anorexic patient with obsessive compulsive disorder, showed up at therapy sessions with her journal pages detached from her journal and inserted in plastic pockets in a binder. It took a number of weeks for her to be able to accept the procedure of working in her journal without detaching and rearranging the pages. They did not need to be separated, even if mistakes were made. Cindy came to learn that entries could follow sequentially and reflect changing styles and themes in an uncomplicated way, even though it was preset.

And after treatment, I encourage patients to make sure that their kits don't have anything missing from them, so they can be ready to journal at home right away. I have also enjoyed presenting new empty journals to patients for the 'home stretch'. The 'home journal' need not be less significant than the one completed during treatment time. I find that it is used on three main occasions. First, at times of stress: worries and concerns can be posted and confronted. Second, to alleviate boredom: doodling, collaging and playing with words can help time pass more productively and quickly. Third, at times of difficulty: it is important to look back and remember how far we have come.

It is also curious to note any differences between sessional work and journalling entries made out of group time. Initially shyer and/or more chronically ill group members, as well as those in individual treatment, may be a little bolder in their journals. As time goes on, differences appear to even out.

CHAPTER II

Resources on Eating Disorders and Art Therapy

The list of resources here is not intended to be all-inclusive. It highlights particular references and associations that have been helpful in writing this book and for my clinical practice, as well as recommendations from those who are experienced in the fields of arts therapies and eating disorders.

Just as the number of eating disorders sufferers is on the increase, so too are the number of publications, associations and treatment centres concerned with them. And I should also like to caution that, particularly in the case of treatment centres, no responsibility can be taken here in terms of success and appropriateness. Camilla Connell (1998) stresses that after viewing artwork created, it is realized that a person's mood cannot necessarily be judged by outward appearances. Thus, similarly, it is wise to check with local and regional eating disorders associations and government healthcare bodies for recommendations, updates and testimonials.

1. Books and book chapters

Eating disorders

Ambramson, E. (1993) *Emotional Eating: A Practical Guide to Taking Control.* New York: Macmillan.

Brown, C. and Karin, J. (eds) (1993) *Consuming Passions: Feminist Approaches to Weight Preoccupation and Eating Disorders.* Toronto: Second Story Press.

Bruch, H. (1987) *The Golden Cage.* London/New York: RKP.

Crisp, A. (1980) *Anorexia Nervosa: Let Me Be.* London: Academic Press.

Fallon, P., Katzman, M.A. and Wooley, S.C. (1994) *Feminist Perspectives on Eating Disorders.* New York: Guilford Press.

Garner, D. and Garfinkel, P. (eds) (1985) *Handbook of Psychotherapy for Anorexia Nervosa and Bulimia.* New York: Guilford Press.

McCleod, S. (1981) *The Art of Starvation*. London: Virago.

Orbach, S. (1978) *Fat is a Feminist Issue*. London: Hamlyn.

Roth, G. (1992) *When Food is Love: Exploring the Relationship between Eating and Intimacy*. USA: Plume.

Schmidt, U. and Treasure, J. (1993) *Getting Better Bit(e) by Bit(e): A Survival Kit for Sufferers of Bulimia Nervosa and Binge Eating Disorders*. East Sussex: Lawrence Erlbaum.

Yager, J., Guirtsman, H.G. and Edelstein, C.K. (eds) (1992) *Special Problems in Managing Eating Disorders*. Washington: American Psychiatric Press.

Yates, A. (1991) *Compulsive Exercise and the Eating Disorders*. New York: Brunner/Mazel Publishers.

Arts therapies and eating disorders

Dokter, D. (ed) (1994) *Arts Therapies and Clients with Eating Disorders: Fragile Board*. London: Jessica Kingsley Publishers.

Fleming, M.M. (1989) 'Art therapy and anorexia: Experiencing the authentic self.' In L.M. Hornyack and E.K. Baker (eds) *Experiential Therapies for Eating Disorders*. New York: Guilford Press.

Hornyack, L.M. and Baker, E.K. (eds) (1989) *Experiential Therapies for Eating Disorders*. New York: Guilford Press.

Levens, M. (1995) *Eating Disorders and Magical Control of the Body: Treatment through Art Therapy*. London: Routledge.

Morenoff, A. and Sobol, B. (1989) 'Art therapy in the long-term psychodynamic treatment of bulimic women.' In L.M. Hornyack and E.K. Baker (eds) *Experiential Therapies for Eating Disorders*. New York: Guilford Press.

Murphy, J. (1984) 'The use of art therapy in the treatment of anorexia nervosa.' In T. Dalley (ed) *Art as Therapy: An Introduction to the Use of Art as a Therapeutic Technique*. London and New York: Tavistock/Routledge.

Schaverien, J. (1994) 'The picture as a transactional object in the treatment of anorexia.' In D. Dokter (ed) *Arts Therapies and Clients with Eating Disorders: Fragile Board*. London: Jessica Kingsley Publishers.

Woodall, C. and Anderson, A.E. (1989) 'The use of metaphor and poetry therapy in the treatment of the reticent subgroup of anorectic patients.' In L.M. Hornyack and E.K. Baker (eds) *Experiential Therapies for Eating Disorders*. New York: Guilford Press.

Art therapy and arts therapies

Circlot, J.E. (1962) *A Dictionary of Symbols (Diccionario de Simbolos Tradicionales)*. Sage, J. (transl.). London: Routledge and Kegan Paul.

Connell, C. (1998) *Something Understood: Art Therapy in Cancer Care*. London: Wrexham Publications.

Cooper, J.C. (1978) *An Illustrated Encyclopaedia of Traditional Symbols*. London: Thames and Hudson.

Dalley, T. (ed) (1984) *Art as Therapy: An Introduction to the Use of Art as a Therapeutic Technique*. London and New York: Tavistock/Routledge.

Kaye, C. and Blee, T. (eds) (1997) *The Arts in Health Care: A Palette of Possibilities*. London: Jessica Kingsley Publishers.

Kramer, E. (1979) *Childhood and Art Therapy*. New York: Schocken Books.

Landgarten, H.B. (1981) *Clinical Art Therapy: A Comprehensive Guide*. New York: Brunner/Mazel.

Makin, S.R. (1994) *A Consumer's Guide to Art Therapy: For Prospective Employers, Clients, and Students*. Springfield, IL: Charles C. Thomas.

Makin, S.R. (1998) *Poetic Wisdom: Revealing and Healing*. Springfield, IL: Charles C. Thomas.

Malchiodi, C.A. (1998) *Understanding Children's Drawings*. New York: Guilford Press.

McNiff, S. (1981) *The Arts and Psychotherapy*. Springfield, IL: Charles C. Thomas.

McNiff, S. (1986) *Educating the Creative Arts Therapist*. Springfield, IL: Charles C. Thomas.

Naumburg, M. (1987) *Dynamically Oriented Art Therapy: Its Principles and Practices*. Chicago: Magnolia Street Publishers.

Rainer, T. (1978) *The New Diary: How to Use a Journal for Self-Guidance and Expanded Creativity*. Los Angeles: Jeremy P. Tarcher.

Rubin, J.A. (1984) *Child Art Therapy*, 2nd edn. London: Van Nostrand Reinhold.

Rubin, J.A. (1984) *The Art of Art Therapy*. New York: Brunner/Mazel.

Wadeson, H. (1980) *Art Psychotherapy*. New York: John Wiley and Sons.

Wadeson, H. (1987) *The Dynamics of Art Psychotherapy*. New York: John Wiley and Sons.

Wadeson, H., Durkin, J. and Perach, D. (1989) *Advances in Art Therapy*. New York: John Wiley and Sons.

Waller, D. (1993) *Group Interactive Art Therapy: Its Use in Training and Treatment*. London: Routledge.

Waller, D. and Gilroy, A. (1992) *Art Therapy: A Handbook*. Buckingham: Open University Press.

2. Journals and journal articles

Journals: Eating disorders

European Eating Disorders Review (four issues per year): John Wiley & Sons, New York.

The International Journal of Eating Disorders (eight issues per year): John Wiley & Sons, New York.

Wiley Journals, 605 Third Avenue, New York, NY 10158, USA. (Tel: 212-850-6009; fax: 212-850-6052)

Journals: Arts therapies

Art Therapy. Journal of the American Art Therapy Association (four issues per year): Mundelein, IL.

Inscape. The Journal of the British Association of Art Therapists (two issues per year): London.

Journal of Poetry Therapy (four issues per year): Human Sciences Press, New York.

The Arts in Psychotherapy (five issues per year): Elsevier Science, New York.

The Canadian Art Therapy Association Journal (two issues per year): Mississauga, Ontario.

Further information about these journals can be obtained from the associations producing them (as listed below, p.190).

Articles: Eating disorders

Batal, H., Johnson, M., Lehman, D., Steele, A. and Mehler, P.S. (1998) 'Bulimia: A primary care approach.' *Journal of Women's Health 7*, 2, 211–220.

Mehler, P.S., Gray, M.C. and Schulte, M. (1997) 'Medical complications of anorexia nervosa.' *Journal of Women's Health 6*, 5, 533–541.

Articles: Eating disorders / body image and the arts therapies

Dosamantes, I. (1992) 'Body-image: Repository for cultural idealizations and denigrations of the self.' *The Arts in Psychotherapy 19*, 4, 257–267.

Franko, D.L. (1993) 'The use of a group meal in the brief group therapy of bulimia nervosa.' *International Journal of Group Psychotherapy 43*, 2, 237–242.

Gillespie, J. (1996) 'Rejection of the body in women with eating disorders.' *The Arts in Psychotherapy 23*, 2, 153–161.

Hendel, A.F. and Levick, M.R. (Introduction and Postscript) (1992) 'Reflections: To Hell and halfway back.' *Art Therapy. Journal of the American Art Therapy Association 9*, 2, 96–102.

Kaslow, N.A. and Eicher, V.W. (1988) 'Body image therapy: A combined creative arts therapy and verbal psychotherapy approach.' *The Arts in Psychotherapy 15,* 177–188.

Kessler, K. (1994) 'Study of the diagnostic drawing series with eating disordered patients.' *Art Therapy. Journal of the American Art Therapy Association 11,* 2, 116–118.

Levens, M. (1987) 'Art therapy with eating disordered patients.' *Inscape,* Summer, 2–7.

Luzzatto, P. (1994) 'Anorexia nervosa and art therapy: The "double trap" of the anorexic patient.' *The Arts in Psychotherapy 21,* 2, 139–143.

Makin, S.R. (1994) 'Art therapy on an inpatient eating disorders programme: Breaking new ground at a large Toronto teaching hospital.' *The Canadian Journal of Art Therapy,* Summer, 26–36.

Matto, H.C. (1997) 'An integrative approach to the treatment of women with eating disorders.' *The Arts in Psychotherapy 24,* 4, 347–354.

Mindell, D. (1980) 'Anorexia nervosa.' *The Arts in Psychotherapy 7,* 53–60.

Naitove, C.E. (1986) 'Life's but a walking shadow. Treating anorexia and bulimia.' *The Arts in Psychotherapy 13,* 107–119.

Place, F. (1994) 'A tale of eating: Writing as a pathway out of an eating disorder.' *Journal of Poetry Therapy 7,* 4, 189–195.

Simonds, S.L. (1992) 'Sexual abuse and body image: Approaches and implications for treatment.' *The Arts in Psychotherapy 19,* 289–293.

Ticen, S. (1987) 'Feed me ... Cleanse me ... Sexual trauma projected in the art of bulimics.' *American Journal of Art Therapy 7,* 1, 17–21.

Waller, C.S. (1992) 'Art therapy with adult female incest survivors.' *Art Therapy 9,* 3, 135–138.

Waller, D. (1981) 'Art therapy in the treatment of eating disorders.' Unpublished paper. Goldsmiths' College, University of London, UK.

Wood, M. (1996) 'Art therapy and eating disorders: Theory and practice in Britain.' *British Journal of Art Therapy 1,* 13–19.

Articles: Arts therapies

Fink, P.J. (1988) 'The importance of the creative arts therapist in psychiatric treatment.' *The Arts in Psychotherapy 15,* 175–176.

Huet, V. (1997) 'Challenging professional confidence: Arts therapies and psychiatric rehabilitation.' *Inscape 2,* 1, 14–19.

Malchiodi, C.A. (1992) 'Editorial. Writing about art therapy for professional publications.' *Art Therapy 9,* 2, 62–64.

McNeilly, G. (1983) 'Directive and non-directive approaches in art therapy.' *The Arts in Psychotherapy 10,* 211–219.

McNeilly, G. (1984) 'Directive and non-directive approaches in art therapy.' *British Journal of Art Therapy 10*, 7–12.

Parker Lewis, P. (1992) 'The creative arts in transference/countertransference relationships.' *The Arts in Psychotherapy 5*, 317–323.

Phillips, J. (1992) 'Collaboration with one's client.' *The Arts in Psychotherapy 19*, 295–298.

Ulman, E. (1986) 'Variations on a Freudian theme: 3 art therapy theorists.' *American Journal of Art Therapy 24*, 4, 125–134.

Ulman, E. (1992) 'Art therapy: Problems of definition.' *The American Journal of Art Therapy 30*, 70–74.

Ulman, E. (1992) 'Innovation and aberration.' *The American Journal of Art Therapy 30*, 98.

Ulman, E. (1992) 'Therapy is not enough: The contribution of art to general hospital psychiatry.' *American Journal of Art Therapy 30*, 89–97.

Ulman, E. and Levy, B. (1992) 'Art therapists as diagnosticians.' *American Journal of Art Therapy 30*, 117–118.

Wadeson, H. (1986) 'The influence of art making on the transference relationship.' *Art Therapy*, July, 81–88.

Waller, D.E. (1992) 'Different things to different people: Art therapy in Britain – A brief survey of its history and current development.' *The Arts in Psychotherapy 9*, 87–92.

Wilson, L. (1985) 'Symbolism and art therapy: Symbolism's role in the development of ego functions.' *American Journal of Art Therapy 23*, February, 79–88.

3. Associations, organizations and related publications

For eating disorders

Academy for Eating Disorders, Montefiore Medical School, Adolescent Medicine, 111 East 210th Street, Bronx, NY 10467, USA. (Tel: 718-920-6782) (for eating disorders professionals).

Eating Disorders Association (EDA), 1st Floor, Wensum House, 103 Prince of Wales Road, Norwich NR1 1DW, UK. (Youthline: (01603) 765050; helpline: (01603) 621414; website: www.gurney.org.uk/eda/; e-mail: eda@netcom.co.uk)

'Statistics regarding eating disorders' (information sheet).

Eating Disorders Awareness and Prevention (EDAP), 603 Stewart Street, Suite 803, Seattle, WA 98101, USA. (Tel: 206-382-587; information line: 800-931-2237; fax: 206-292-9890; website: http://members.aol.com/edapinc)

'Statistics: Eating disorders and their precursors' (information sheet).

National Eating Disorder Information Centre (NEDIC), c/o Toronto General Hospital, 200 Elizabeth Street, CW 2–332, Toronto, Ontario. (Tel: 416-340-4156; fax: 416-340-4736; website: www.nedic.on.ca)

'Guide for family and friends of a person experiencing food and weight problems' (one-page handout).

'Understanding and overcoming an eating disorder: A resource kit for those with anorexia nervosa and bulimia nervosa.'

For the arts therapies

International Expressive Arts Therapy Association (IEATA), PO Box 320152, San Francisco, CA 94132, USA. (Tel: 415-522-8959)

The American Art Therapy Association, Inc., 1202 Allanson Road, Mundelein, IL 60060, USA. (Tel: 847-949-6064; website: http://www.arttherapy.org; e-mail: arttherapy@ntr.net)

The British Association of Art Therapists, Mary Ward House, 5 Tavistock Place, London WC1H 9SN, UK. (Tel: 0171 383 3774; fax: 0171 387 5513)

The Canadian Art Therapy Association, 6–2400 Dundas Street West, Suite 601, Mississauga, Ontario, Canada L5K 2R8. (Tel: 905-469-9442; website: http://www.ican.net/~phansen/pages/CATA.html)

The National Association for Poetry Therapy, Box 280, 5505 Connecticut Avenue N.W., Washington DC 20015, USA. (Tel: 202-966-2536; website: http://www.poetrytherapy.org; e-mail: rdaniel@his.com)

4. Internet websites and links

For eating disorders:

http://www.mirror-mirror.org/resack.htm (Canadian site)

http://www.something-fishy.org/ed-4.htm (American site)

http://www.something-fishy.org/amazon.htm (for books on eating disorders)

For art therapy:

http://home.ican.net/~phansen/index.html (Canadian site)

Conclusion

1. Art therapy's magic

The arts therapies are effective on a number of levels. First, for the association-making opportunities that they present. Second, for the meditative processes that they induce: occasions for self-soothing and play. Third, for the insights, clarifications and possibilities for change that may be created in reviewing and discussing artwork. Subjects such as far-back memories and special occasions that come round too often for all of us manage to be revealed in art content, even if not touched in other groups.

When I used to paint extensively in watercolours, I would talk about the magic of that medium, how the white areas would get covered up by surprising leakages of colour, just because I let them be. The more I work with the arts therapies, the more I learn that, beyond gentle guiding and witnessing, I need to let patients be.

The magic of art therapy happens for me in what patients say, unprompted, about their experience or product, or both. They talk of how the session worked or didn't work for them, for reasons about which I may or may not have thought. The patients, creators of incredible artefacts, hold the key to them, and are the only ones who can provide access to their worlds and accompanying particularities.

2. Responses of patients with eating disorders to arts therapies

Traditionally, eating-disordered populations generate towards arts and craft activities and are usually very comfortable with them. Even for the inexperienced artist, art media offer a non-threatening way to explore, play and mess; and manageable new skills can help build self-esteem. The opportunity to make tangible visualizations is very helpful, since images are distorted routinely by eating-disordered patients.

Even the most resistant have come to ameliorate their opinions about the benefits of the arts therapies over time. Anne was a 24-year-old anorexic patient who had had two admissions to the eating disorders programme at the hospital and several art therapy experiences. She wrote up an account of her art therapy experiences, dividing them into four phases:

- *Phase 1* (month one, in hospital, admission one): pencils, rulers, lots of words, collaging, real things (not abstract).

- *Phase 2* (the next three months, in hospital, admission one): larger pieces and a personal quota of five per week.

- *Phase 3* (the following four months at home): on own initiative, more inventive.

- *Phase 4* (the following four months, in hospital, admission two): moving from 'she' to 'I' expressions.

She then wrote a summary of her changing feelings concerning art therapy:

Today, I admit to its benefits. When I began, however, I was clearly more of a sceptic. It was my belief, when first introduced to art therapy, that it centred on choices based on opinions and false interpretations. Through a long process, I have come to realize that art indeed opened my eyes to that which I refused to see.

Initially, I rejected all suggestions and would ridicule those who portrayed it as helpful. Fights would erupt, from my side, with every suggestion made to me to use specific or different media. I failed to realize the importance of not sticking to that which comforts me rather than that which may reveal emotions. I was determined to make light of this 'serious' element of my recovery.

As I reflect back on my work, it is difficult not to notice the tremendous change I have gone through, both as a recovering anorexic as well as an adult accepting advice from those who know. In an attempt to look more closely at the barriers to change that I have overcome, I compare the artwork which I produced during my second admission, when more ready and able to change, to the artwork done in my first admission, when it was clear to everyone that I did not really wish to recover.

Moving from my depressive thoughts in black and white, I have shifted to more variety of colours and media. I find it difficult to choose a favourite, as all media are challenging to me and often reveal that which I forbid myself to verbally express. As one who is fond of words and writing, I found that the more reliant I became on my art (to express thoughts), the less words I felt obliged to use in explanation of it, and the more able I was to talk in the first as opposed to third person (going from 'she' to 'I').

It is a difficult task to single out a piece of work as liked or disliked. I have learned to deviate from my perfectionist personality which focused on the product to focusing on the process and the message the art tries to send to me. So long as thought and time was devoted to my work, it was successful in relaying hidden emotions. I needed this challenge in my road to recovery. I consider my art to be as important as my written journals. Perhaps viewing my work in the future will reveal to me more than I know today about myself.

Moving beyond eating disorders, and formal art therapy, I have found that many patients have become so engaged in the art-making process during their art therapy treatment opportunities that art-making for therapy and otherwise becomes an important part of their lives afterwards. Marjorie, the 30-year-old anorexic and abused patient whose artwork features prominently in Chapter 7, took up photography after her discharge. Marjorie is still not recovered, but manages to maintain herself in a 'holding pattern'. Her adventures with the camera, about which she is very proud, give her a sense of enthusiasm and 'life' that she is unable to get anywhere else. And, I have been interested to note, most of the subjects she focuses on tend to be solitary objects: a lone feather on a beach, or a boat tied up on the shore.

Also, some former patients even express an interest in finding out more about art therapy, that they may consider a career involving it. Rachel, whose creative journal entries are included in Chapter 6, was back at an out-of-town university a couple of months after discharge and in a psychology class writing an essay on art therapy. So, she contacted me for some assistance. She also informed me at that time about the cartoon character she had developed for a student newspaper, whose genesis had been in her creative journal. The trademark feature in the art journal, an oversized mouth, was also dominant in the cartoon character version.

3. Integrating art therapy in multidisciplinary team settings

In the multidisciplinary team setting, the arts therapist acts as a supportive team member, offering extra professional expertise and helping with the synthesis of information. When verbal techniques are not enough, the arts therapist facilitates visual responses from patients that confirm or shed new light on social histories and symptomatologies. When presentations of patients' artwork are included at team meetings, it can feel like the patient is actually there, her artwork representing herself. Also, any changes or manifestations of concern made in other areas, as described by team members who use verbal techniques, appear to be mirrored in the artwork.

Susan Wooley, a prominent eating disorders verbal therapist, in her foreword to the book *Experiential Therapies for Eating Disorders* (Wooley 1989), talks of her early experience with expressive modalities:

> In learning to speak another language I entered their world of uncertainty. Stripped of my words, I had no choice but to be more real, more spontaneous. There was no well-worn script to refer to, only the immediacy of the moment. This, in turn, led me to more innocent, real and profound connections to my patients. (p.vii)

In the US and Britain, practitioners from other mental health modalities increasingly affirm the arts therapies, as evinced in the creation of more positions and budgets for them. In Canada, unfortunately, limited knowledge about the arts therapies, the competitiveness and insecurities of practitioners from more traditional disciplines, as well as healthcare budget cut-backs, often impede advancement of the arts therapies. The result is poorer clinical outcome for difficult-to-treat patient groups, such as those with eating disorders. Impasses occur when other treatment team members recognize the effectiveness of the arts therapies, but are unfamiliar with their theories and techniques, some of which may sometimes be better than other aspects of multidisciplinary team programming.

As an arts therapist, I have no desire to do any more than my position should entail; but I have still met with frustrations. I agree with June Murphy when she describes art therapy as providing another dimension in the treatment of anorexics, allowing opportunities for lines of communication to be opened, in ways that patients were not previously able to express. I also agree with her when she insists that 'success' with anorexic patients is not forthcoming by using art therapy techniques alone: the art therapist cannot work in isolation but needs to liaise with an experienced multidisciplinary team (Murphy 1984).

Timing is everything, and it is hard for systems to remedy what may be described by some as 'growing pains'. For eating disorders programmes to work, no matter how good the individual groups are (arts therapies included), there must be mutual respect for, and understanding of, all team members' approaches and disciplines. Otherwise success is not guaranteed for patients or therapists and the programme. Murphy also believes that art therapy should not be isolated as a form of treatment with eating-disordered

patients: its efficacy with this population can only be evaluated effectively
when the contributions of other therapists and treatment methods, experienced simultaneously, are taken into account as well. Val Huet, a British art
therapist, warns that, when arts therapists are not able to be present at team
meetings, rounds and reviews, good communications can be put at risk. She
acknowledges, however, that other staff are usually aware that arts therapists
are mostly part-timers, making regular and unpaid attendance difficult for
them (Huet 1997).

Then, there is the problem of arts therapies-related jargon, which can
make arts therapists seem 'aloof and unapproachable'. It is important to note
here that the jargons of other disciplines, such as medicine and psychology,
may be taken for granted as well. Huet also draws attention to a correlation
between the amount of personal contact other professionals have with the
arts therapist and the understanding of her input. And since work with
clients is directly influenced by the quality of co-operation between staff,
Huet confesses that 'acknowledging problems and doubts takes courage'
(p.19).

4. Finally ... and thank you

Ideally, the arts therapies are best engaged in a safe space, with a therapist
trained in these modalities serving as guide. However, if an arts therapist is
not available, when an individual needing treatment is so inclined, an activity
such as creative journalling can be a helpful, safe, soothing and clarifying
experience to engage in alone.

I would also like to highlight my concern here that even as we enter the
new millennium, a majority of clinicians still exercise natural tendencies to
put themselves on pedestals, particularly when giving case presentations. I
recommend that the more there can be a shift away from their rigid, dry,
second- and third-person accounting to using first-person patient-centred or
client-centred expressive reporting, the closer to the truth and effective
treatment we can come.

So, in closing, it is very important for me to emphasize heart-felt
appreciation to the patients who have enthusiastically said it as it is (however
painful) and allowed their first-hand accounts and images to be printed in
this book. Without their support, faith and recognition in the possibilities to
provide relief and recovery for eating disorders through art therapy, this
book could not have come into being. At the points when I doubted my
capacity to complete this project, I looked back at my patients' notes – their

authenticity – knowing the meaningfulness and possibilities for growth they would impart for others, particularly if in similar conditions.

And finally, I would now like to encourage clinicians to go on to this book's companion, *Therapeutic Art Directives and Resources: Activities and Initiatives for Individuals and Groups* (Makin 1999). Here you will find myriad ways to develop your own practice, not only with patients with eating disorders, but with other populations also. There is so much to be shared in this area that the second book is not only a natural follow-on text, but a necessary addition to the general literature on art therapy.

Bibliography

Alpers, J. (1997) 'Book review: D. Dokter (ed) *Arts Therapies and Clients with Eating Disorders: Fragile Board.*' *The Arts in Psychotherapy 24*, 1, 105–109.

American Psychiatric Association (1994) *Diagnostic and Statistical Manual of Mental Disorders*, 4th edition. Washington, DC: American Psychiatric Association.

Anderson, A.E. (1998) Paper presented at the Eighth New York International Conference on Eating Disorders. April 24–26, New York.

Batal, H., Johnson, M., Lehman, D., Steele, A. and Mehler, P.S. (1998) 'Bulimia: A primary care approach.' *Journal of Women's Health 7*, 2, 211–220.

Cleghorn, J.M. and Lee, B.L. (1991) *Understanding and Treating Mental Illness: The Strengths and Limits of Modern Psychiatry*. Toronto: Hongrefe and Huber.

Connell, C. (1998) *Something Understood: Art Therapy in Cancer Care*. London: Wrexham Publications.

Dokter, D. (ed) (1994) *Arts Therapies and Clients with Eating Disorders: Fragile Board*. London: Jessica Kingsley Publishers.

Dosamantes, I. (1992) 'Body-image: Repository for cultural idealizations and denigrations of the self.' *The Arts in Psychotherapy 19*, 4, 257–267.

Dubowski, J.K. (1992) 'Editorial.' *The Arts in Psychotherapy 19*, 79–81.

EDA (1997) (Eating Disorders Association, UK) 'Statistics Regarding Eating Disorders.' Information sheet.

EDA (1999) 'Accurate statistics.' E-mail message to Susan Makin, March 15.

EDAP (1999) 'Statistics: Eating Disorders and their Precursors.' Information Sheet.

Edwards, B. (1979) *Drawing on the Right Side of the Brain*. Los Angeles: J.P. Tarcher.

Fleming, M.M. (1989) 'Art therapy and anorexia: Experiencing the authentic self.' In L.M. Hornyack and E.K. Baker (eds) *Experiential Therapies for Eating Disorders*. New York: Guilford Press.

Gardner, H. (1983) *Frames of Mind: The Theory of Multiple Intelligences*. New York: Basic Books.

Gillespie, J. (1996) 'Rejection of the body in women with eating disorders.' *The Arts in Psychotherapy 23*, 2, 153–161.

Goleman, D. (1995) *Emotional Intelligence: Why It Can Matter More Than IQ.* New York: Bantam Books.

Huet, V. (1997) 'Challenging professional confidence: Arts therapies and psychiatric rehabilitation.' *Inscape 2*, 1, 14–19.

Kaslow, N.A. and Eicher, V.W. (1988) 'Body image therapy: A combined creative arts therapy and verbal psychotherapy approach.' *The Arts in Psychotherapy 15*, 177–188.

Katzman, M. (1998) Paper presented at the Eighth New York International Conference on Eating Disorders. April 24–26, New York.

Kaye, C. and Blee, T. (eds) (1997) *The Arts in Health Care: A Palette of Possibilities*. London: Jessica Kingsley Publishers.

Lee, S. (1998) Paper presented at the Eighth New York International Conference on Eating Disorders. April 24–26, New York.

Levens, M. (1987) 'Art therapy with eating disordered patients.' *Inscape*, Summer, 2–7.

Lowenfeld, V. and Brittain, W.L. (1987) *Creative and Mental Growth*, 8th edition. New York and London: Collier Macmillan.

Luzzatto, P. (1994) 'Anorexia nervosa and art therapy: The "double trap" of the anorexic patient.' *The Arts in Psychotherapy 21*, 2, 139–143.

Makin, S.R. (1998) *Poetic Wisdom: Revealing and Healing*. Springfield, IL: Charles C. Thomas.

Malchiodi, C.A. (1998) *Understanding Children's Drawings*. New York: Guilford Press.

Marcus, M. (1998) Paper presented at the Eighth New York International Conference on Eating Disorders. April 24–26, New York.

Matto, H.C. (1997) 'An integrative approach to the treatment of women with eating disorders.' *The Arts in Psychotherapy 24*, 4, 347–354.

McNiff, S. (1981) *The Arts and Psychotherapy*. Springfield, IL: Charles C. Thomas.

Mehler, P.S., Gray, M.C. and Schulte, M. (1997) 'Medical complications of anorexia nervosa.' *Journal of Women's Health 6*, 5, 533–541.

Mitchell, D. (1980) 'Anorexia nervosa.' *The Arts in Psychotherapy 7*, 53–60.

Morenoff, A. and Sobol, B. (1989) 'Art therapy in the long-term psychodynamic treatment of bulimic women.' In L.M. Hornyack and E.K. Baker (eds) *Experiential Therapies for Eating Disorders*. New York: Guilford Press.

Murphy, J. (1984) 'The use of art therapy in the treatment of anorexia nervosa.' In T. Dalley (ed) *Art as Therapy: An Introduction to the Use of Art as a Therapeutic Technique*. London and New York: Tavistock/Routledge.

Naumburg, M. (1950 and 1973) *An Introduction to Art Therapy*. New York: Teachers College Press.

Place, F. (1994) 'A tale of eating: Writing as a pathway out of an eating disorder.' *Journal of Poetry Therapy 7*, 4, 189–195.

Schaverien, J. (1994) 'The picture as a transactional object in the treatment of anorexia.' In D. Dokter (ed) *Arts Therapies and Clients with Eating Disorders: Fragile Board*. London: Jessica Kingsley Publishers.

Stein, D., Luria, A., Glick, D., Yoeli, N., Elizur, A. and Weizman, A. (1998) Paper presented at the Eighth New York International Conference on Eating Disorders. April 24–26, New York.

Ticen, S. (1987) 'Feed me … Cleanse me … Sexual trauma projected in the art of bulimics.' *American Journal of Art Therapy 7*, 1, 17–21.

Treasure, J. (1998) Paper presented at the Eighth New York International Conference on Eating Disorders. April 24–26, New York.

Waller, C.S. (1992) 'Art therapy with adult female incest survivors.' *Art Therapy 9*, 3, 135–138.

Waller, D. (1981) 'Art therapy in the treatment of eating disorders.' Unpublished paper. Goldsmiths' College, University of London, UK.

Walsh, B.T. (1995) Paper presented at 'Eating Disorders '95'. The 2nd London International Conference on Eating Disorders. April 25–27, London.

Wilson, L. (1985) 'Symbolism and art therapy: Symbolism's role in the development of ego functions.' *American Journal of Art Therapy 23*, February, 79–88.

Wood, M. (1996) 'Art therapy and eating disorders: Theory and practice in Britain.' *British Journal of Art Therapy 1*, 13–19.

Woodall, C. and Anderson, A.E. (1989) 'The use of metaphor and poetry therapy in the treatment of the reticent subgroup of anorectic patients.' In L.M. Hornyack and E.K. Baker (eds) *Experiential Therapies for Eating Disorders.* New York: Guilford Press.

Wooley, S. (1989) 'Foreword.' In L.M. Hornyack and E.K. Baker (eds) *Experiential Therapies for Eating Disorders.* New York: Guilford Press.

Subject Index

Author Index

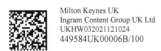

Milton Keynes UK
Ingram Content Group UK Ltd.
UKHW032021121024
449584UK00006B/100